THE DOCTOR'S GUIDE
TO CRITICAL APPRAISAL
SECOND EDITION

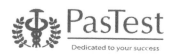

PasTest
Dedicated to your success

THE DOCTOR'S GUIDE TO CRITICAL APPRAISAL
SECOND EDITION

Dr Narinder Kaur Gosall
BSc (Hons) PhD

Director, Superego Cafe Limited

Dr Gurpal Singh Gosall
MA MB BChir MRCPsych

Consultant General Adult Psychiatrist,
Lancashire Care NHS Foundation Trust
Director, Superego Cafe Limited

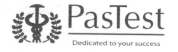

PasTest
Dedicated to your success

Egerton Court
Parkgate Estate
Knutsford
Cheshire WA16 8DX

Telephone: 01565 752000

First edition 2006, Second edition 2009

ISBN: 1 905635 567
ISBN: 978 1 905635 566

A catalogue record for this book is available from the British Library.

The information contained within this book was obtained by the authors from reliable sources. However, while every effort has been made to ensure its accuracy, no responsibility for loss, damage or injury occasioned to any person acting or refraining from action as a result of information contained herein can be accepted by the publisher or the authors.

PasTest Revision Books and Intensive Courses

PasTest has been established in the field of undergraduate and postgraduate medical education since 1972, providing revision books and intensive study courses for doctors preparing for their professional examinations.

Books and courses are available for:

Medical undergraduates, MRCGP, MRCP Parts 1 and 2, MRCPCH Parts 1 and 2, MRCS, MRCOG Parts 1 and 2, DRCOG, DCH, FRCA, Dentistry.

For further details contact:

PasTest, Freepost, Knutsford, Cheshire WA16 7BR

Tel: 01565 752000   **Fax: 01565 650264**

www.pastest.co.uk   **enquires@pastest.co.uk**

Text prepared by Carnegie Book Production, Lancaster
Printed by Athenaeum Press Ltd, Gateshead, Tyne & Wear

CONTENTS

About the authors   viii

Introduction to the 2nd edition   ix

Introduction to the 1st edition   x

Acknowledgements   xi

Introducing critical appraisal   xiii

SECTION A – FIRST IMPRESSIONS   **1**

The journal   3

Organisation of the article   5

The clinical question   7

Primary hypothesis   10

SECTION B – METHODOLOGY   **11**

Overview of methodology   13

Observational descriptive studies   15

Observational analytical studies   17

Experimental studies   20

Other types of study   24

The hierarchy of evidence   28

Research pathway   30

Populations and samples   32

Bias   34

Confounding factors   39

The placebo effect   44

Restriction   46

Matching   47

Randomisation   48

Concealed allocation   51

Blinding   53

Endpoints   56

Validity   58

Reliability   60

SECTION C – RESULTS   63

Types of data   65

Measuring data   67

Describing data from one sample   69

Inferring population results from samples   74

Epidemiological data   78

Risks and odds   82

Comparing samples – the null hypothesis   87

Comparing samples – statistical tests   94

Non-inferiority and equivalence trials   101

Correlation and regression   103

Intention-to-treat analysis   107

Interim analysis   112

Systematic reviews and meta-analyses   113

Heterogeneity and homogeneity   117

Publication bias   121

SECTION D – APPLICABILITY   125

Applicability   127

SECTION E – CHECKLISTS   129

Checklists   131

Aetiological studies   132

Diagnostic or screening studies   133

Treatment studies   141

Prognostic studies   143

Economic studies   147

Qualitative research   153

SECTION F – CRITICAL APPRAISAL IN PRACTICE   155

Health information resources   157

Presenting at a journal club   163

Taking part in an audit meeting   166

Working with pharmaceutical representatives   168

Further reading   172

Answers to self-assessment exercises   175

A final thought   184

Index   185

Dedicated to our son, Dilip

ABOUT THE AUTHORS

Dr Narinder Kaur Gosall BSc (Hons) PhD
Director, Superego Cafe Limited

Narinder Gosall studied in Liverpool and gained a PhD in neuropathology after investigating the role of the phrenic nerve in sudden infant death syndrome and intrauterine growth retardation. After working as a university lecturer she joined the pharmaceutical industry. She worked in a variety of roles, including as a Medical Liaison Executive and as a Clinical Effectiveness Consultant for Pfizer Limited. She has extensive experience in teaching critical appraisal skills to healthcare professionals and is an international speaker on the subject. She is the editor of the online course at www.criticalappraisal.com.

Dr Gurpal Singh Gosall MA MB BChir MRCPsych
Consultant General Adult Psychiatrist, Lancashire Care NHS
Foundation Trust
Director, Superego Cafe Limited

Gurpal Gosall studied medicine at the University of Cambridge and Guy's and St Thomas's Hospitals, London. He worked as a Senior House Officer in Psychiatry in Leeds before working as a Specialist Registrar in the Manchester rotation. He now works as a Consultant Psychiatrist based in Clitheroe, Ribble Valley. He has had a long-standing interest in teaching and runs a popular website for psychiatrists, Superego Cafe, at www.superego-cafe.com.

Learning the skill of critical appraisal is like learning a foreign language – wherever you start, you come across unfamiliar words and concepts. However, persistence pays off and, like speaking a foreign language, the earlier it is mastered and the more it is used, the easier critical appraisal becomes.

Unfortunately many clinicians have never been taught critical appraisal skills and many are not even aware that books and courses exist to help them. They sit in awe in academic meetings as their peers discuss the pros and cons of journal articles. Rather than taking the lead in implementing research findings, many clinicians wait for others to guide them.

We wrote the first edition of this book three years ago to explain critical appraisal to the busy clinician. Based on our teaching experience, we took a unique back-to-basics approach that provided a logical and comprehensive review of the subject. This new edition expands on that earlier work with updated information and more help with difficult topics.

We hope that by reading this book you will start reading clinical papers with more confidence. The language of evidence-based medicine is not as foreign as you might think.

NKG, GSG

2009

INTRODUCTION TO THE 1ST EDITION

One of the attractions of a career in medicine is that it is forever advancing. Hardly a day goes by without a new discovery about a disease process or an exciting innovation in the management of an illness. This book aims to help doctors who want to practice medicine at the leading edge. It is not enough simply to read the latest journal articles. Doctors need to examine critically the research laid before them and decide which evidence to take to the bedside. They need to lead their teams to higher standards of patient care based on robust evidence about what works and what doesn't work.

The skill of evaluating research is so valuable that there is no room for academic snobbery. We hope that this book is a refreshing change to the reader, explaining the principles of critical appraisal in an easy-to-read format. We have tried to make the subject appear as simple as possible – because it *is* simple. If, after reading this book, the reader is better able to evaluate the next journal article he or she reads, we will have done our job. Enjoy.

NKG, GSG

2006

ACKNOWLEDGEMENTS

We would like to express our thanks to Cathy Dickens (Commissioning Editor) and Fiona Power (Technical Editor) and the rest of the PasTest team for their help and support with this book. Thanks also to Elizabeth Kerr, formerly of PasTest, who worked on the first edition.

We thank our teachers and colleagues for generously sharing their knowledge and for providing guidance. We are also indebted to all the healthcare professionals who have attended our critical appraisal courses and provided us with comments and helpful suggestions about our teaching materials.

We would like to express our gratitude to our families, who inspired us and gave us unconditional support during the writing of this book. In addition, a special thank-you goes to Guj for his constant belief and encouragement during our endeavours.

July 2009

INTRODUCING CRITICAL APPRAISAL

Scenario 1

Dr Jones was annoyed. Six months ago, he was given a clinical paper by a pharmaceutical sales representative about a new treatment for high blood pressure. The results of the trial were certainly impressive. On the basis of the evidence presented, he prescribed the new tablet to all his hypertensive patients. Instead of the expected finding that four out of every five patients would lower their blood pressure, only one out of every ten of his patients improved. He decided to present the article in the hospital journal club, as he himself couldn't see where in the study the mistake lay. He then hoped to confront the sales representative for wasting his time and the hospital's money.

Every year, thousands of clinical papers are published in the medical press. The vast range of topics reflects the complexity of the human body, with studies all fighting for our attention. Separating the 'wheat from the chaff' is a daunting task for doctors, such that many rely on others for expert guidance.

In 1972, the publication of Archie Cochrane's *Effectiveness and Efficiency: Random Reflections on Health Services*[1] made doctors realise how unaware they were about the effects of healthcare. Archie Cochrane, a British epidemiologist, went on to set up the Cochrane Collaboration in 1992. It is now an international organisation, committed to producing and disseminating systematic reviews of health-care interventions. Bodies such as the Cochrane Collaboration have made the lives of doctors much easier, but the skill of evaluating evidence should be in the arsenal of every doctor.

Evidence-based medicine

Evidence-based medicine is the phrase used to describe the process of practising medicine based on a combination of the best available research evidence, our clinical expertise and patient values. As such, evidence-based medicine has had a tremendous impact on improving healthcare outcomes since its widespread adoption in the early 1990s.

The most widely quoted definition of evidence-based medicine is that it is *'the conscientious, explicit and judicious use of current best evidence in making decisions about the care of the individual patient'*[2]. The practice of evidence-based medicine comprises five steps, shown in **Table 1**.

1   Cochrane AL. *Effectiveness and efficiency: random reflections on health services*. London, Royal Society of Medicine Press, 1999.
2   Sackett DL, Richardson WS, Rosenberg W, Haynes RB. *Evidence-based medicine: how to practice and teach evidence-based medicine*. London, Churchill Livingstone, 1997.

EVIDENCE-BASED MEDICINE – THE FIVE STEPS		
1	Question	Formulate a precise, structured clinical question about an aspect of patient management
2	Evidence	Search for the best evidence with which to answer the question
3	Critical appraisal	Evaluate the evidence, critically appraising the evidence for its validity, impact and applicability
4	Application	Apply the results to clinical practice, integrating the critical appraisal with clinical expertise and with patients' circumstances
5	Implementation & monitoring	Implement and monitor this whole process, evaluating the effectiveness and efficacy of the whole process and identify ways to improve them both for the future

Table 1 Evidence-based medicine – the five steps

Evidence-based medicine begins with the formulation of a clinical question, such as 'What is the best treatment for carpal tunnel syndrome?' This is followed by a search of the medical literature looking for answers to the question. The evidence gathered is appraised and the recommendations from the best studies are applied to patients. The final step, which is often overlooked, is to monitor any changes and repeat the process.

Although evidence-based medicine has led to a more consistent and uniform approach to clinical practice, it does not mean that clinicians practice identically. Clinicians vary in their expertise, so that not all the recommendations from clinical research can be followed. For example, the evidence may suggest an intramuscular injection is the best treatment for a condition but the clinician may not have been trained to safely administer the treatment. Also, patients differ in the interventions they find acceptable – some patients may prefer not to have an injection. Finally, the lack of resources may also restrict the choices available, particularly for new and expensive interventions.

Critical appraisal
In the process of evidence-based medicine, why do we need a step on critical appraisal? Why not take all results at face value and apply all the findings to clinical practice? The first reason is that there may be conflicting conclusions drawn from different studies. Secondly, real-life medicine rarely follows the restrictive environments in which clinical trials take place. To apply, implement

and monitor evidence, we need to ensure that the evidence we are looking at can be translated into our own clinical environments.

Critical appraisal is just one step in the process of evidence-based medicine, allowing doctors to assess the research found and decide which research will have a clinically significant impact on their patients. Critical appraisal allows doctors to exclude research that is too poorly designed to inform medical practice. By itself, critical appraisal does not lead to improved outcomes. It is only when the conclusions drawn from critically appraised studies are applied to everyday practice and monitored that the outcomes for patients improve.

Critical appraisal assesses the validity of the research and statistical techniques employed in studies, and generates clinically useful information from them. It seeks to answer two major questions:

- Does the research have **internal validity** – to what extent do the results from the study reflect the true results by taking into consideration the study design and methodology?

- Does the research have **external validity** – to what extent can the results from the study be generalised to a wider population?

As with most subjects in medicine, it is not possible to learn about critical appraisal without coming across jargon. Wherever we start, we will come across words and phrases we do not understand. In this book we try to explain critical appraisal in a logical and easy-to-remember way. Anything unfamiliar will be explained in due course.

Efficacy and effectiveness

Two words that are useful to define now are 'efficacy' and 'effectiveness'. They are sometimes used interchangeably, but they have different meanings and consequences in the context of evidence-based medicine.

Efficacy describes the impact of interventions under optimal (trial) conditions.

Effectiveness is a different but related concept, describing whether the interventions have the intended or expected effect under ordinary (clinical) circumstances.

Efficacy shows that internal validity is present. Effectiveness shows that external validity (generalisability) is present.

The contrast between efficacy and effectiveness studies was first highlighted 30 years ago by Schwartz and Lellouch[3]. Efficacy studies usually have the aim of seeking regulatory approval for licensing. The interventions in such studies tend to be strictly controlled and compared with placebo interventions. The

3   Schwartz D, Lellouch J. Explanatory and pragmatic attitudes in therapeutical trials. *Journal of Chronic Diseases* 1967, 20, 637–48.

people taking part in such studies tend be a selective 'eligible' population. In contrast, effectiveness studies tend to be undertaken for formulary approval. Dosing regimens tend to be more flexible and compared with interventions already being used. Almost anyone is eligible to enter such trials.

It is not always easy and straightforward to translate the results from clinical trials (efficacy data) to uncontrolled clinical settings (effectiveness data). There are many factors which mean that results achieved in everyday practice do not always mirror an intervention's published efficacy data. The efficacy of an intervention is nearly always more impressive than its effectiveness.

Scenario 1 revisited

The journal club audience unanimously agreed that the double-blind randomised controlled trial was conducted to a high standard. The methodology, the analysis of the results and the conclusions drawn could not be criticised. When Dr Jones queried why his results were so different, the chairman of the journal club commented, "My colleague needs to understand the difference between efficacy data and his effectiveness data. I assume his outpatient clinic and follow-up arrangements are not run to the exacting standards of a major international trial! May I suggest that, before criticising the work of others, he should perhaps read a book on critical appraisal?"

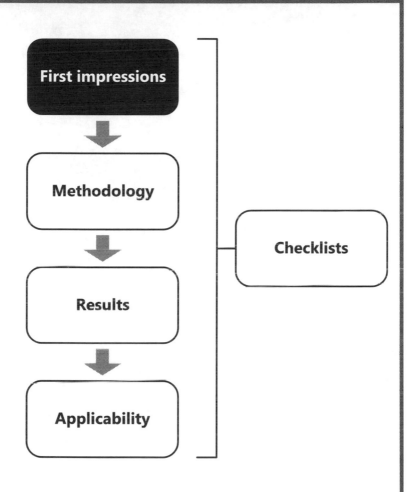

Not all journals are equal. Some journals are more prestigious than others. There may be many reasons for such prestige, including a long history in publishing, affiliation with an important medical organisation or a reputation for publishing important research. It is important to know in which journal an article was published – but remember, poor articles are published in even the best journals, and vice versa.

Peer-reviewed journals

A **peer-reviewed** journal is a publication that requires each submitted article to be independently examined by a panel of experts who are non-editorial staff of the journal. To be considered for publication, articles need to be approved by the majority of peers. The process is usually anonymous, with the authors not knowing the identities of the peer reviewers. In double-blind peer review, neither the author nor the reviewers know each other's identities. Anonymity aids the feedback process.

The peer review process forces authors to meet certain standards laid down by researchers and experts in that field. Peer review makes it more likely that mistakes or flaws in research are detected before publication. As a result of this quality assurance, peer-reviewed journals are more highly regarded than non-peer-reviewed journals.

There are disadvantages to the peer review process. First, it adds a delay between the submission of an article and its publication. Secondly, the peer reviewers may guess the identity of the author(s), particularly in small specialised fields, impairing the objectivity of their assessments. Thirdly, revolutionary or unpopular conclusions can face opposition within the peer review process, leading to preservation of the status quo.

Journal impact factor

A **journal impact factor** provides a means of evaluating or comparing the performance of a journal relative to others in the same field. It ranks a journal's importance by the number of times articles within that journal are cited by others. A higher frequency of citation implies that the journal is found to be useful to others, suggesting that the research published in the journal is valuable. Impact factors are calculated annually by the Institute for Scientific Information and published in the Journal Citation Reports. In 2007 the *New*

England Journal of Medicine had an impact factor of 52.589 and the *British Medical Journal* had an impact of 9.723.

The journal impact factor[4] is a measure of the frequency with which the average article in a journal has been cited in a particular year. The **impact factor** is the number of citations in the current year to articles published in the two previous years, divided by the total number of articles published in the two previous years. In critical appraisal, the journal impact factor cannot be used to assess the importance of any one article, as the impact factor is not specific to that article.

The **immediacy index** is another way of evaluating journals from the Institute for Scientific Information. It measures how often articles published in a journal are cited within the same year. This is useful for comparing journals specialising in cutting-edge research.

A journal can improve its impact factor by improving accessibility to its articles and publicising them more widely. In recent years there have been significant improvements in web-based access to journals and now some journals publish research articles online before they appear in print. Many journals issue press releases highlighting research findings and send frequent email updates to subscribers. A rise in the percentage of review articles published in a journal can also boost its impact factor.

4   *Journal citation reports (JCR)*. Philadelphia, USA. Thomson Institute for Scientific Information, 2005. JCR provides quantitative tools for ranking, evaluating, categorising and comparing journals.

ORGANISATION OF THE ARTICLE

The majority of published articles follow a similar structure.

Title of the article: This should be concise and informative, but sometimes an attention-grabbing title is used to attract readers to an otherwise dull paper. The title can influence the number of people reading the article, which might in turn lead to increased citations.

Author(s): This should allow you to see if the authors have the appropriate academic and professional qualifications and experience. The institutions at which the authors work may also be listed and can increase the credibility of the project if they have a good reputation for research in this field.

Abstract: This summarises the research paper, briefly describing the reasons for the research, the methodology, the overall findings and the conclusions made. Reading the abstract is a quick way of getting to know the article, but the brevity of the information given means that it is unlikely to reveal the strengths and weaknesses of the research. If the abstract is of interest to you, you must go on to read the rest of the article. Never rely on an abstract alone to inform your medical practice!

Introduction: This explains what the research is about and why the study was carried out. A good introduction will include references to previous work related to this subject matter and describe the importance and limitations of what is already known.

Method: This gives detailed information about how the study was actually carried out. Specific information is given on the study design, the population of interest, how the sample of the population was selected, the interventions offered and which outcomes were measured and how they were measured.

Results: This shows what happened to the individuals studied. It may include raw data and explain the statistical tests used to analyse the data. The results may be portrayed in tables, diagrams and graphs.

Conclusion / discussion: This discusses the results in the context of what is already known about the subject area and the clinical relevance of what has been found. It may include a discussion on the limitations of the research and suggestions on further research.

Conflicts of interest / funding: Articles should be published on their scientific merit. A conflict of interest is any factor that interferes with the objectivity of research findings. Conflicts of interest can be held by anyone involved in the research project, from the formulation of a research proposal through to its publication, including authors, their employers, sponsoring organisation, journal editors and peer reviewers. Conflicts of interest can be financial (eg research grants, honoraria for speaking at meetings), professional (eg member of an organisational body) or personal (eg relationship with the journal's editor). Ideally, authors should disclose conflicts of interest when they submit their research work. **A conflict of interest does not necessarily mean that the results of a study are void.**

Ileal-lymphoid-nodular hyperplasia, non-specific colitis, and pervasive developmental disorder in children

A J Wakefield et al., Lancet, 351, 28 February 1998

This study raised the possibility of a link between the measles, mumps and rubella vaccine (MMR) given to children in their second year of life and inflammatory bowel disease and autism. This was widely reported by the media. The MMR scare reduced vaccination rates to 80% nationally, leading to a loss of herd immunity and measles outbreaks returned to the UK. Later it was revealed that the lead author was being funded through solicitors seeking evidence to use against vaccine manufacturers and he also had a patent for a single measles vaccine at the time of the study. Ten of the study's 13 authors later signed a formal retraction[1]. The editor of the Lancet said the research study would never have been published if he had known of a serious conflict of interest.

1   Murch SH, Anthony A, Casson DH, et al. 'Retraction of an interpretation'. Lancet 2004, 363, 750.

THE CLINICAL QUESTION

Scenario 2
Dr Green, a General Practitioner, smiled as she read the final draft of her research paper. Her survey of 50 patients with fungal nail infections demonstrated that more than half of them had used a public swimming pool in the month before infection. She posted a copy of the paper to her Public Health Consultant, proposing she submit the article to the Journal of Public Health.

A common misconception is that the study design is the most important determinant of the merits of a clinical paper. As soon as the words 'randomised controlled trial' appear, many doctors assume that the study is of great value and the results can be applied to their own medical practice. If this approach was true, then there would be no need for any other type of study.

The critical appraisal of a paper must begin by looking at the clinical question that is at the heart of the paper. **The clinical question determines which study designs are appropriate.**

- One clinical question can be answered by a number of study designs.
- No single study design can answer all clinical questions.

The clinical question
There are five broad categories for clinical questions, as shown in **Table 2**.

CLINICAL QUESTION	CLINICAL RELEVANCE AND POSSIBLE STUDY DESIGNS
Diagnosis	How valid and reliable is a diagnostic test? What does the test tell the doctor? Example: case–control study
Aetiology/causation	What caused the disorder and how is this related to the development of the illness? Example: randomised controlled trial, case–control study, cohort study
Therapy	Which treatments do more good than harm compared with an alternative treatment? Example: randomised controlled trial, systematic review, meta-analysis
Prognosis	What is the likely course of a patient's illness? What is the balance of the risks and benefits of treatments? Example: cohort study, longitudinal survey
Cost-effectiveness	Which intervention is worth prescribing? Is newer treatment X worth prescribing compared to older treatment Y? Example: economic analysis

Table 2 The different types of clinical question

Usually, broad questions such as 'How do I treat diabetes mellitus?' and 'What causes bowel cancer?' are easy to understand. These questions are looking for general information.

The acronym 'PICO', explained in **Table 3**, can help to break down more complex questions which seek more specific answers. 'PICO' phrases questions in a way that also directs the search to relevant and precise answers.

P	Patient or Problem	Describe your patient and their problem
I	Intervention	Describe the main intervention, exposure, test or prognostic factor under consideration
C	Comparison	In the case of treatment, describe a comparative intervention. A comparison is not always needed.
O	Outcomes	Describe what you hope to achieve, measure or affect.

Table 3 Introducing PICO

An example of PICO is shown in **Table 4**.

P	Patient or Problem	In a middle-aged male with schizophrenia ...
I	Intervention	... what is the likelihood of olanzapine ...
C	Comparison	... compared to haloperidol ...
O	Outcomes	... producing a greater improvement in symptoms?

Table 4 An example of PICO

Scenario 2 revisited

Dr Green's colleague was less enthusiastic about the findings. He wrote, "Interesting though the results are, your chosen study design shows merely an association between swimming pools and fungal nail infections. I think you wanted to know whether a causative relationship exists. I'm afraid a cross-sectional survey cannot answer that question. Before you panic the Great British public, may I suggest you go back to the drawing board and, based on your question, choose a more appropriate study design?"

PRIMARY HYPOTHESIS

The type of clinical question determines the types of study that will be appropriate. In the methodology, the researcher must specify how the study will answer the clinical question. This will usually involve stating a hypothesis and then explaining how this hypothesis will be proven or not proven. The hypothesis is usually the same as or closely related to the clinical question.

A study should, ideally, be designed and powered to answer one well-defined hypothesis.

If there is a secondary hypothesis, its analysis needs to be described in the same way as that for the primary hypothesis. The protocol should include details of how the secondary outcomes will be analysed. Ideally, further exploratory analyses should be identified before the completion of the study, and there should be a clear rationale for the reason and value of such analyses.

Finally, not all studies are designed to test a hypothesis. Some studies, such as case reports or qualitative studies, can be used to generate hypotheses.

Subgroup analysis

Data dredging is a problem in research studies and sometimes it can result in researchers testing for everything but only reporting the significant results.

Performing many subgroup analyses has the effect of greatly increasing the chance that at least one of these comparisons will be statistically significant, even if there is no real difference (type 1 error). For example, where several factors may influence outcome (eg sex, age, ethnicity, smoking status) the risk of false-positive results is high. As a result, conclusions can be misleading. Deciding on subgroups after the results are available can also lead to bias.

Multiple-hypothesis testing on the same set of results should be avoided. Subgroup analyses should be restricted to a minimum and subgroup analyses should be pre-specified in the methodology whenever possible. Any analyses suggested by the data should be acknowledged as exploratory for generating hypotheses.

Self-assessment exercise 1

A study fails to meet its primary hypothesis but it is statistically significant for its secondary and tertiary hypotheses. What conclusions will you draw?

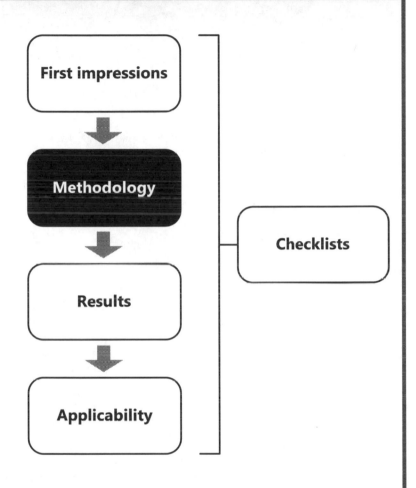

OVERVIEW OF METHODOLOGY

In a clinical paper the methodology employed to generate the results is described. Generally, the following questions need to be answered:

- What is the clinical question that needs to be answered?
- What is the study design?
- How many arms are there in the study and how do they differ?
- Who are the subjects? How are they recruited and allocated to the different arms?
- What is being measured and how?

Any shortcoming in the methodology can lead to results which do not reflect the truth. If clinical practice is changed based on these results, patients could be harmed.

The researchers may highlight methodological problems in the discussion part of the paper but the onus is still on the reader to appraise the methodology carefully. Thankfully most problems fall into two categories: bias and confounding factors. If the methodology is found to be totally flawed, the results become meaningless and cannot be applied to clinical practice no matter how good they are.

Researchers employ a variety of techniques to make the methodology more robust, such as matching, restriction, randomisation and blinding. In the following chapters it will become clear why these techniques are used.

Reading the methodology is therefore an active process in which strengths and weaknesses are identified.

Introducing study designs
The type of clinical question determines the types of studies that will be appropriate. Study designs fall into three main categories:

1. **Observational descriptive studies** – the researcher reports what has been observed in a sample.

2. **Observational analytical studies** – the researcher reports the similarities and differences observed between two or more samples.

3. **Experimental studies** – the researcher intervenes in some way with the experimental group and reports any differences in the outcome between this experimental group and a control group where no intervention or a different intervention was offered.

In the next four chapters, examples of study designs will be given. The advantages and disadvantages of different designs may include references to terms which we have not yet covered. (**Figure 5** on page 27 is a flowchart which can be used to decide study type.)

Terms used to describe studies

Longitudinal: Deals with a group of subjects at more than one point in time.

Cross-sectional: Deals with a group of subjects at a single point in time (ie a snapshot in time).

Prospective: Deals with the present and the future (ie looks forward).

Retrospective: Deals with the present and the past (ie looks back).

Ecological: A population or community is studied, giving information at a population rather than an individual level. Ecological studies can use pre-recorded data.

Pragmatic: Trials may be described as either explanatory or pragmatic. Explanatory trials tend to measure efficacy. Pragmatic trials measure effectiveness because the trials take place in ordinary clinical locations such as outpatient clinic departments. The results of these trials are considered to be more reflective of everyday practice as long as the patients selected are representative of the patients who will receive the treatment. Often a new treatment is compared with a standard treatment rather than with a placebo. Pragmatic trials tend to be difficult to control, difficult to blind, and there are difficulties with excessive drop-outs.

Cluster: In these trials, groups or clusters of people are randomly assigned to study groups instead of individual patients. These trials can be useful to evaluate the delivery of health services.

OBSERVATIONAL DESCRIPTIVE STUDIES

In observational descriptive studies, the researcher describes what has been observed in a sample. Nothing is done to the subjects in the sample. There is no control group for comparison. These studies are useful for generating hypotheses that can be tested using other study designs.

Case report

A single patient is studied. Case reports are easy to write, but they tend to be anecdotal and cannot usually be repeated. They are also prone to chance association and bias. Their value lies in the fact that they can be used to generate a hypothesis.

The Medicines and Healthcare products Regulatory Agency's 'Yellow Card Scheme' is an example of case reports on patients who have suffered suspected adverse drug reactions. Yellow Card reports are evaluated each week to find possible previously unidentified hazards and other new information on the side-effects of medicines.

Case series

A group of patients are studied. Case series are useful for rare diseases.

There are hardly any journals devoted to publishing case reports and case series alone. These studies are more likely to be found in poster presentations in conferences and as letters or rapid responses in journals. Case reports and case series are low down in the hierarchy of evidence but are useful to identify new diseases, symptoms and signs, aetiological factors, associations, treatment approaches and prognostic factors.

A famous case series was published as a letter in the *Lancet* in 1961[1], in which WG McBride wrote, "*Sir, Congenital abnormalities are present in approximately 1.5% of babies. In recent months I have observed that the incidence of multiple severe abnormalities in babies delivered of women who were given the drug thalidomide during pregnancy, as an antiemetic or as a sedative, to be almost 20%. Have any of your readers seen similar abnormalities in babies delivered of women who have taken this drug during pregnancy?*" The link with congenital abnormalities led to the withdrawal of thalidomide from the market.

1   McBride WG. Thalidomide and congenital abnormalities. *Lancet* 1961, 2, 1358.

OBSERVATIONAL ANALYTICAL STUDIES

In observational analytical studies, the researcher reports the similarities and differences observed between subjects in two or more groups.

Case–control study

Subjects who have the outcome variable are compared with individuals who don't have the outcome variable, to find out what risk factors the groups have been exposed to in the past (**Figure 1**). The researcher hopes to show that subjects with the outcome variable are more likely to have been exposed to one or more risk factors compared with the control group. Case–control studies are also known as 'case comparison' or 'retrospective case–control' studies. They are used to investigate the causes of outcomes. They are particularly valuable in the study of rare diseases and in situations where there is a long time interval between exposure and outcome.

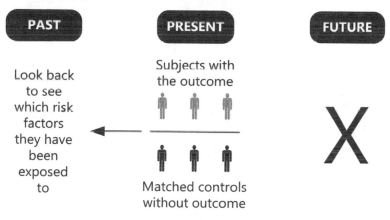

Figure 1 Case–control study design

Case–control studies are usually quick and cheap to do, as few subjects are required, but it may be difficult to recruit a matching control group. The major problem with case–control studies is the need to rely on recall and records to determine which risk factors the subjects have been exposed to. They are also not good for studying rare exposures, as too many subjects with the outcome would be required. The temporal relationship between exposure and outcome may be difficult to establish.

Smoking and carcinoma of the lung; preliminary report.
R. Doll, A. Bradford Hill. *British Medical Journal* 1950, 221, 739–48
A case–control study in which patients who had suspected lung, liver or bowel cancers were asked about past exposure to risk factors, including smoking. Those with lung cancer were confirmed as smokers, and those who were given the all-clear were non-smokers.

Cohort study

A group of subjects are followed up to see how the likelihood of an outcome differs between groups with and without exposure to a risk factor (**Figure 2**). The researcher hopes to show that subjects exposed to a risk factor are more likely to get the outcome compared with the control group. Cohort studies are used to investigate the consequences of exposure to risk factors, so they are able to answer questions about aetiology and prognosis. Unlike case-control studies, cohort studies are suitable for studying rare exposures. They can assess temporal relationships and multiple outcomes. They can also give a direct estimation of disease incidence rates.

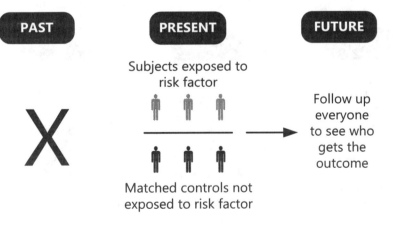

Figure 2 Cohort study design

Cohort studies are unsuitable for studying rare outcomes, as the number of subjects required to detect the rare outcome would be large. There can also be a long time interval from exposure to the development of the outcome. These studies are therefore expensive to set up and maintain. Selection bias becomes a problem if subjects drop out of the study. Confounding factors can also be a problem. Blinding is difficult and there is no randomisation.

The mortality of doctors in relation to their smoking habits: a preliminary report
R. Doll, A. Bradford Hill. *British Medical Journal* 1954, 1451–5
A cohort study which examined the relationship between smoking and lung cancer. 24,389 doctors were divided into two groups depending on whether or not they were exposed to the risk factor (smoking). 29 months later, an examination of the cause of 789 deaths revealed a significant and steadily rising mortality from deaths due to lung cancer as the amount of tobacco smoked increased.

Cohort studies are also known as 'prospective' or 'follow-up' studies.

Sometimes a study is described as a **retrospective cohort study**. This sounds paradoxical but a retrospective cohort design simply means that the researcher identified a cohort study already in progress and added another outcome of interest. This saves the researcher time and money by not having to set up another cohort from scratch.

Association or causation?

Observational analytical studies are often used to show the association between exposure and outcome. Deciding if a causative relationship exists is made easier by using Sir Austin Bradford Hill's nine considerations for assessing the question, 'When does association imply causation?'[5]

- **Strength:** Is the association strong and large enough that we can rule out other factors?

- **Consistency:** Have the results been replicated by different researchers, in different places, circumstances and times?

- **Specificity:** Is the exposure associated with a very specific disease?

- **Temporality:** Did the exposure precede the disease?

- **Biological gradient:** Are increasing levels of exposure associated with an increased risk of disease?

- **Plausibility:** Is there a scientific mechanism that can explain the causative relationship?

- **Coherence:** Is the association consistent with the natural history of the disease?

- **Experimental evidence:** Is there evidence from other randomised experiments?

- **Analogy:** Is any association analogous to any previously proved causal association?

5   Austin Bradford Hill. 'The Environment and Disease: Association or Causation?' *Proceedings of the Royal Society of Medicine*, 58 (1965), 295–300.

SECTION B METHODOLOGY

EXPERIMENTAL STUDIES

In experimental studies, the researcher intervenes in some way with the experimental group and reports any differences in the outcome between this experimental group and a control group in whom no intervention or a different intervention was offered.

Open trial

All the subjects in the study are given the same treatment. In the absence of a control group, these studies are cheap and easy to perform.

Controlled trial

Subjects in the study are given one of two treatments. The absence of randomisation can, however, introduce biases in the results.

Randomised controlled trial

The gold standard design for studying treatment effects. Subjects in the study are randomly allocated a treatment, which minimises selection bias and can equally distribute confounding factors between the treatment arms depending on the randomisation strategy. The use of blinding reduces observation bias. Randomised controlled trials (RCTs) are a reliable measure of efficacy and allow for meta-analyses, but they are difficult, time-consuming and expensive to set up. There may be ethical problems in giving different treatments to the groups and there is a problem with selection bias.

Crossover trial

All the subjects receive one treatment and then switch to the other treatment halfway through the study (**Figure 3**). Crossover trials are often used to study rare diseases where the lack of subjects would make a conventional trial under-powered.

The crossover design has another advantage. A researcher in a treatment study needs to ensure that the subjects in the two arms are similar, so that any difference in outcome can be attributed to the presence or absence of treatment. In a crossover study the subjects are their own controls, so matching is almost perfect. The word 'almost' is used because usually in research studies the results in the experimental arm are compared with the control arm at the same point in time. In a crossover design, the comparison takes place at different time points. This may be a problem if something changes that means dissimilar conditions exist at the two time points.

The researcher must also ensure that there are no carry-over effects from the first intervention that could impact on how well the subjects do with the second intervention. Carry-over effects may be caused by long half-lives and discontinuation effects. These problems can be reduced by using wash-out periods. The order in which the interventions are given can also be important.

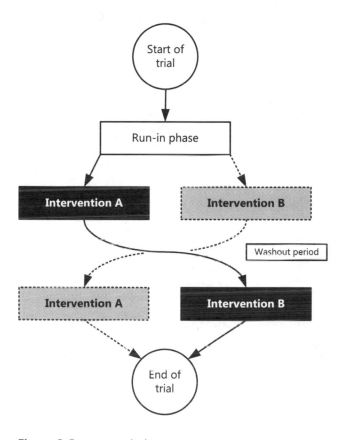

Figure 3 Crossover study design

n-of-1 trial

In an 'n-of-1' trial a single subject is studied and receives repeated courses of the active drug and placebo in a random order. The subject reports on his progress regularly. This can establish effectiveness in a particular subject, as it can reveal whether clinical improvement occurs only at the time of being in receipt of the active drug.

The CONSORT statement

First published in *Journal of the American Medical Association* in August 1996, the Consolidated Standard of Reporting Trials (CONSORT) statement introduced a set of recommendations to improve the quality of randomised controlled trial reports[6]. This checklist is summarised in **Table 5**.

SECTION OF PAPER	DESCRIPTION
Title & abstract	How participants were allocated to interventions
Introduction	Scientific background and explanation of rationale
Methods	
Participants	Eligibility criteria for participants
Interventions	Details of the interventions for each group
Objectives	Specific objectives and hypotheses
Outcomes	Clearly defined primary and secondary outcome measures
Sample size	How sample size was determined
Randomisation – sequence generation	Method used to generate the random allocation sequence
Randomisation – allocation concealment	Method used to implement the random allocation sequence
Randomisation – implementation	Who generated the allocation sequence, who enrolled participants, and who assigned participants to their groups
Blinding	Whether or not participants, those administering the interventions, and those assessing the outcomes were blinded to group assignment

6   Moher D, Schulz KF, Altman DG. The CONSORT statement: revised recommendations for improving the quality of reports of parallel-group randomised trials. *Lancet* 2001, 357, 1191–4.

SECTION OF PAPER	DESCRIPTION
Statistical methods	Statistical methods used to compare groups for primary outcome(s)
Results	
Participant flow	Flow of participants through each stage
Recruitment	Dates defining the periods of recruitment and follow-up
Baseline data	Baseline demographic and clinical characteristics of each group
Numbers analysed	Number of participants in each group and whether the analysis was by 'intention to treat'
Outcomes and estimation	For each primary and secondary outcome, a summary of results for each group, and the estimated effect size and its precision
Ancillary analyses	Address multiplicity by reporting any other analyses performed
Adverse events	All important adverse events or side-effects in each intervention group
Discussion	
Interpretation	Interpretation of the results
Generalisability	Generalisability (external validity) of the trial findings
Overall evidence	General interpretation of the results in the context of current evidence

Table 5 The CONSORT checklist

The Standards for Quality Improvement Reporting Excellence (SQUIRE) Group have also published guidelines to improve standards[7].

7   Davidoff F, Batalden P, Stevens D, Ogrine G, Mooney SE, Publication guidelines for quality improvement studies in health care: evolution of the SQUIRE project. BMJ 2009, 338, a3152.

OTHER TYPES OF STUDY

Audit

Aspects of service provision are assessed against a gold standard, which can be a national guideline, a local protocol, or generally accepted best practice. Sometimes it is necessary to devise a gold standard in the absence of a published one.

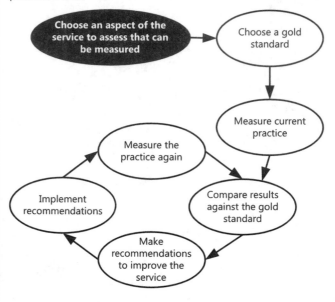

Figure 4 The audit cycle

Data on the service are collected and compared with the gold standard. A change is then implemented in the running of the service and the audit cycle is completed by another collection of data (**Figure 4**).

Audits give information on the effectiveness of services. However, they are resource-hungry and take clinicians away from clinical work.

Survey

A group of subjects are questioned. Surveys can identify patterns and help to plan service provision. Surveys cannot distinguish between cause and effect.

In a **qualitative survey** opinions are elicited from a group of subjects, with the emphasis on the subjective meaning and experience. Such studies can be used to study complex issues. The inquiry can be via interviews, focus groups and participant observation. However, it can be difficult to get information, record it and analyse the subjective data.

In a **cross-sectional survey**, subjects are questioned for the presence of risk factors and outcomes. They are useful for establishing prevalence. They establish association, not causality. Such surveys are cheap, simple and are ethically safe. The groups can be unequal, confounders might be asymmetrically distributed and recall bias is a problem. Large numbers of subjects are usually required.

Economic analysis

This type of study assesses the cost and/or utilities of intervention. Such analyses help to prioritise services, but it is difficult to remain objective because assumptions have to be made.

Systematic review and meta-analysis

A systematic review attempts to access and review systematically all of the pertinent articles in the field. A meta-analysis combines the results of several studies and produces a quantitative assessment.

Self-assessment exercise 2
What types of studies are suggested by the following statements?

1. Patients with ankle injuries who are seeing a physiotherapist are questioned about the type of trainers they wear in order to investigate the relationship between running shoes and susceptibility to ankle injuries. The answers are compared with those of healthy people.

2. Builders exposed to asbestos on a demolition site are seen regularly, to detect any adverse consequences.

3. A consultant physician investigates how many patients newly referred to the outpatient clinic are seen within 16 weeks of the date of referral.

4. Patients with chronic lower back pain are randomly given one of two treatments and assessed regularly.

5. Residents in a leafy suburb are questioned about their opinions on whether planning permission should be given for a new psychiatric medium-secure unit in the neighbourhood.

6. The Primary Care Trust investigates whether to allocate funds originally set aside for an obesity clinic towards a new treatment for bowel cancer instead.

Self-assessment exercise 3

1. You have developed a blood test for detecting meningitis. How will you set up a study to see if your test is any good?

2. You have developed a new treatment for patients with anorexia nervosa. How will you set up a study to see if your new treatment is any good?

3. You suspect that smoking cannabis leads to the onset of schizophrenia. How will you set up a study to see if this is true?

4. You think that outpatients who are diagnosed with a frozen shoulder will never return to work. How will you set up a study to see if your suspicions are right?

Self-assessment exercise 4

1. What are the advantages and disadvantages of a crossover design compared with a traditional randomised controlled trial?

2. How do cohort studies differ from case–control studies? Which is preferred for investigating the effect of rare exposures? Which is preferred for investigating the cause of rare outcomes?

3. What restriction is imposed on the choice of topics that you as a clinician can audit?

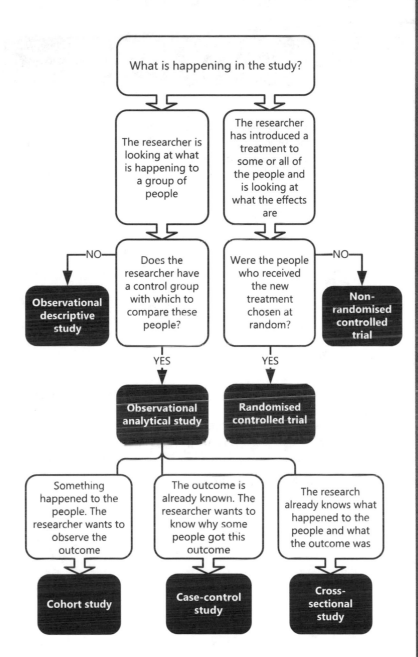

Figure 5 Distinguishing between study types — summary

THE HIERARCHY OF EVIDENCE

There is a well-established hierarchy of research methodologies. The hierarchy is based on the premise that the study designs differ in their ability to predict what will happen to patients in real life. The studies at the top of the hierarchy carry more weight than studies lower down because their evidence is of a higher grade.

Systematic review / meta-analysis
Randomised controlled trial
Non-randomised controlled trial
Cohort studies
Case–control studies
Cross-sectional surveys
Case series
Case report
Expert opinion
Personal communication

Studies that carry greater weight are not necessarily the best in every situation and are unlikely to be appropriate for all situations. For example, a case report can be of great importance, even though in terms of the hierarchy of studies a case report normally carries the least weight. Also note that the hierarchy is for guidance only; not all studies using the same design are of equal quality.

The NHS Centre for Reviews and Dissemination (CRD) has published its view of the hierarchy of evidence (**Table 6**)[8].

8   University of York, NHS Centre for Reviews and Dissemination. *Undertaking systematic reviews of research on effectiveness: CRD guidelines for those carrying out or commissioning reviews.* CRD Report Number 4 (2nd edition), March 2001.

STUDY DESIGN HIERARCHY	
Level	**Description**
1	Experimental studies (eg RCT with concealed allocation)
2	Quasi-experimental studies (eg experimental study without randomisation)
3	Controlled observational studies 3a Cohort studies 3b Case–control studies
4	Observational studies without control groups
5	Expert opinion based on pathophysiology, bench research or consensus

Table 6 CRD guidelines on the hierarchy of evidence

The National Institute for Clinical Excellence (NICE) also publishes guidance, which is evidence-based[9]. It grades its recommendations in a similar way (Table 7).

STUDY DESIGN HIERARCHY	
Level	**Description**
A	Based on level I evidence (meta-analysis of randomised controlled trials or at least one randomised controlled trial)
B	Based on level II or level III evidence (well-conducted clinical studies but no randomised controlled trials) or extrapolated from level I evidence
C	Based on level IV evidence (expert committee reports or opinions and/ or clinical experience of respected authorities)
GPP	Recommended good practice based on clinical experience of the Guideline Development Group
N	Evidence from NICE technology appraisal guidance

Table 7 Grading of recommendations from NICE

9   NICE website: http://www.nice.org.uk/

RESEARCH PATHWAY

Bringing a drug to the market can take several years and cost hundreds of millions of pounds (**Figure 6**). The developmental process usually begins with the identification of a biological target that is linked with the aetiology of a disease. Compounds are formulated to act on this target. The chosen compound is then transformed and packaged in such a way that it can be administered to patients to give the maximum benefit and the minimum of side-effects. This transformation process involves a series of trials on animals and humans that are subject to the rigorous controls required by the regulatory authorities and local ethics committees.

Clinical trial authorisations are needed for all new products in development. Applications for such authorisations in the United Kingdom are assessed by the medical, pharmaceutical and scientific staff at the Medicines and Healthcare products Regulatory Agency (MHRA), an agency of the Department of Health.

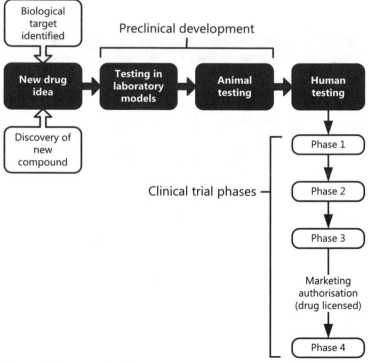

Figure 6 The research pathway

Clinical trial phases
Clinical trials of experimental drugs consist of four phases.

Phase 1 clinical trials
These are the earliest trials in the life of a new drug or treatment. The researchers test a new drug or treatment in a small group of **healthy people** for the first time, to assess its safety, establish a dose range and identify any side-effects. These trials aim to help in the evaluation and understanding of the behaviour of the molecule or compound. The healthy volunteers are normally compensated for the time they are giving up but are not given financial incentives to take part in research.

Phase 2 clinical trials
About seven out of every ten new treatments tested at phase 1 in healthy volunteers proceed to phase 2 trials and are tested on **people with the relevant illness**. At this stage, the study drug or treatment is given to a larger group of people, to assess its effectiveness and safety profile.

Phase 3 clinical trials
At this stage, the study drug or treatment is given to large groups of people in **clinical settings** to make further assessments of its effectiveness, dose range and duration of treatment, and to monitor side-effects. These trials compare the new treatment with the best currently available treatment (the standard treatment).

Providing satisfactory results are gained from phase 3 studies, a drug will get a **marketing authorisation**, which sets out its agreed terms and conditions of use, such as indications and dose range. Even drugs with a high risk-to-benefit ratio may be approved if the drug enhances the quality of life of patients with terminal illnesses, for example.

Phase 4 clinical trials
Phase 4 trials, also known as 'post-marketing surveillance studies', are carried out after a drug has been shown to work, granted a licence and marketed. Information is collected about the benefits and side-effects of the drug in different populations. Data on long-term usage are also collected. These studies involve monitoring the safety of medicines under their usual conditions of use, and can also be carried out to identify any new safety concerns (**hypothesis generating**) and to confirm or refute these concerns (**hypothesis testing**).

POPULATIONS AND SAMPLES

Researchers identify the target population they are interested in. It is rarely feasible to include everyone in the target population in the trial. A sample population is therefore taken and results from this sample are then generalised to the target population (**Figure 7**). The size of the sample population can be determined by a power calculation.

The sample should be representative of the target population it came from. Knowing the **baseline characteristics** of the sample population is important, as it allows doctors to see how closely the subjects match their own patients. Such characteristics can include demographic characteristics, such as age and sex, as well as more fluid variables, such as smoking status. Often these details are given in the form of a table in the research paper.

When we consider the applicability of research findings, we are usually asking firstly whether the sample population in the study is representative of the target population and, secondly, whether our patients match those in the study's target population. If the sample population is unrepresentative or the target population is unlike our own, the research findings might not be applicable to our patients, no matter how good the evidence.

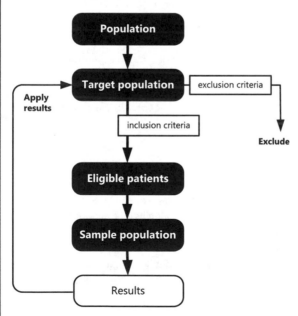

Figure 7 Describing people at the different stages of a study

Inception cohort: A group of patients who are assembled near the onset of the target disorder.

Methods of sampling

There are five common techniques that are used to obtain a sample from a population:

1. **Random sampling:** Every person in the target population has an equal chance of being selected. Random sampling is also known as **representative** and **proportionate** sampling because all groups should be *proportionately represented*.

2. **Systematic sampling:** Every n^{th} member of the target population is selected once the first person has been chosen at random.

3. **Stratified sampling:** Different populations of people are recruited from particular subgroups or strata in the target population. This is achieved by dividing the target population into two or more strata based on one or more characteristics, and sampling each stratum (usually randomly).

4. **Cluster sampling:** The target population is divided into clusters and some of these clusters are exhaustively sampled.

5. **Convenience sampling:** Sampling is done as convenient, often allowing the subject to choose whether or not he/she is sampled. Convenience sampling is the easiest and potentially most dangerous. Often good results can be obtained, but perhaps just as often the data set may be seriously **biased**.

TO SUMMARISE, A GOOD STUDY WILL ...

Describe the target population

Explain how the sample population was recruited

Explain how the sample size was determined

Comment on how well the sample population represents the target population

BIAS

Scenario 3

Dr Pahal, Consultant Plastic Surgeon, was interested in how many patients would use a hospital website to access information about postoperative care. He placed an advertisement in The Times newspaper and recruited 90 people for his survey. He concluded that 70% of patients would definitely visit a hospital website for more information about the management of surgical wounds. He put forward a proposal to the Hospital Board for funding the development of such a website.

Scenario 4

Consultant Psychiatrist, Dr Thomas, had a long-standing interest in the treatment of anxiety disorders. His Clinical Director wanted him to set up a specialist clinic for patients with anxiety disorders, but needed to justify the expense to the Hospital Board. Dr Thomas sent a postal questionnaire to 500 patients of the psychiatry unit, asking them if they had ever been told they had a neurotic disorder. If the answer was 'yes', he asked them to describe the treatments offered and whether they would support the development of a specialist clinic.

Scenario 5

Nurse Smith wanted to illustrate the quality of care provided by her team to patients on a gastroenterology ward. She visited every patient on the day of their discharge home and took them through a questionnaire to rate the quality of the care they received during the hospital stay. She presented the near-perfect results to the matron and asked for a salary increase.

Errors in studies can lead to results that are misleading and conclusions that are wrong. Interventions and treatments can appear more or less beneficial than they actually are. Errors in studies can happen either by chance or through mistakes in the way the study was done.

Bias is used to describe an error (at any stage of the study) that was not due to chance, and therefore it cannot be measured or controlled for statistically. Researchers need to rely on good research design to minimise bias. The presence of bias leads to results in which there is a systematic deviation from the truth.

There are many types of bias. The main types of bias can be listed either at the stage of the study at which they arise or in the broad categories of reporting, selection, performance, observation or attrition bias (**Table 8**).

STAGE OF STUDY	CATEGORIES OF BIAS	EXAMPLES OF BIAS	STRATEGIES TO AVOID BIAS
Literature review	Reporting	Literature search bias	Comprehensive search strategy
		Foreign language exclusion bias	Translation
Recruitment of a sample population	Selection	Sampling bias (researcher): - Berkson bias - Diagnostic purity bias - Neyman bias - Membership bias - Historical control bias	Randomisation Concealed allocation
		Response bias (subjects)	
Running the trial	Performance	Instrument bias Questionnaire bias	Blinding
Collecting data	Observation	Interviewer bias Recall bias Response bias Hawthorne effect	Blinding outcome assessment
Analysing the results	Attrition	Attrition (exclusion) bias	Intention-to-treat analysis

Table 8 The different types of bias

Selection bias

This occurs through the identification and/or recruitment of an unrepresentative sample population. The sample population differs in some significant way from the population that generated the sample population, such that any results and conclusions drawn from the sample population cannot be generalised to the population target. This is a potential problem for all studies.

Selection bias can be further divided into sampling bias, which is introduced by the researchers, or response bias, which is introduced by the study population.

Examples of **sampling bias** include:

- **Berkson (admission) bias:** This arises when the sample population is taken from a hospital setting, but the hospital cases do not reflect the rate or severity of the condition in the population. The relationship between exposure and disease is unrepresentative of the real situation.

- **Diagnostic purity bias:** This arises when co-morbidity is excluded in the sample population, such that the sample population does not reflect the true complexity of cases in the population.

- **Neyman (incidence / prevalence) bias:** This occurs when the prevalence of a condition does not reflect its incidence. Usually this is due to a time gap between the onset of a condition and the actual selection of the study population, such that some individuals with the condition are not available for selection.

- **Membership bias:** This arises when membership of a group is used to identify study individuals. The members of such a group may not be representative of the population.

- **Historical control bias:** This arises when subjects and controls are chosen across time, such that secular changes in definitions, exposures, diseases and treatments may mean that such subjects and controls cannot be compared with one another.

Response bias occurs when individuals volunteer for studies but they differ in some way from the population. The most common reason for such a difference is that the volunteers are more motivated to improve their health and therefore participate more readily and adhere to the trial conditions better. Confusingly, the term 'response bias' can also be used to describe an observation bias (see below).

Performance bias

Performance bias occurs when differences arise in the care that is provided to the subjects in the different arms.

Observation bias

Observation bias occurs as a result of failure to measure or classify the exposure or outcomes correctly. It can be due to the researchers or the subjects.

Examples of observation bias include:

- **Interviewer (ascertainment) bias:** This arises when the researcher is not blinded to the subject's status in the study and this alters the researcher's approach to the subject and the recording of results.

- **Recall bias:** This arises when subjects selectively remember details from the past. This can be particularly important in case–control studies and cross-sectional surveys.
- **Response bias:** This arises in any study in which the subjects are asked questions, if the subjects answer questions in the way they believe the researcher wants them to answer, rather than according to their true beliefs.
- **Hawthorne effect:** This arises when subjects alter their behaviour, usually positively, because they are aware that they are being observed in a study.

Attrition bias

Attrition bias arises when the numbers of individuals dropping out of the study differ significantly in the different arms of the study. Those left at the end of the study may not be representative of the study sample that was randomised at the start.

Scenario 3 revisited

Dr Pahal's proposal was rejected by the Hospital Board. In their conclusions, they commented: "A non-representative sample was used to generate the findings. The population that the hospital serves is dissimilar to that which reads The Times newspaper in a number of respects, including, but not limited to, lower literacy levels and less internet access. Dr Pahal should consider selecting a more representative sample for future proposals, to avoid selection bias."

Scenario 4 revisited

Dr Thomas's survey generated a surprising result, with only 1% of the sample having been diagnosed with a neurotic disorder. His Clinical Director wrote to him, stating that, "Perhaps nowadays not many people are familiar with the term 'neurotic'. The use of the word 'anxiety' may produce different results as it will eliminate observation bias. Please repeat the survey."

Scenario 5 revisited

The matron was less than impressed. She commented, "The results are good but what else did you expect if you asked patients about their views? They're hardly likely to give you negative comments! Perhaps I should ask an independent organisation to survey the patients at home? That will eliminate a response bias. I'm afraid a salary rise cannot be justified at this time. Now get back to work."

Self-assessment exercise 5

For each of the following study protocols, decide if selection and/or observation bias may occur.

1. **Study aim:** To plan the provision of stroke services for elderly patients.
   Proposed method: A cross-sectional survey to discover the prevalence of cerebrovascular accidents by phoning 5000 residents across the city.

2. **Study aim:** To elicit the magnitude of drug problems in the teenage population.
   Proposed method: A survey of teenagers in all the schools in the city, asking them about illicit use of drugs.

3. **Study aim:** To investigate the association between smoking and lung cancer.
   Proposed method: A case–control study of inpatients in a respiratory disease ward in a district general hospital.

4. **Study aim:** To establish the effectiveness of pain relief offered to women during childbirth.
   Proposed method: A questionnaire sent to new mothers asking them about their experience of pain during delivery.

TO SUMMARISE, A GOOD STUDY WILL ...

Explain how the selection process minimised selection bias

Explain what techniques were employed to minimise observation bias

Acknowledge any mistakes or methodological compromises that were made

Make suggestions on how any mistakes can be avoided in future research, if possible

CONFOUNDING FACTORS

Scenario 6

Dr Edwards designed a case–control study to investigate the relationship between alcohol consumption and lung cancer. She recruited 700 people, both healthy controls and lung cancer sufferers, into her study. She questioned each person on their alcohol history. To her surprise she found a significant relationship, showing that alcohol consumption increased the risk of lung cancer, such that the finding was unlikely to have happened by chance alone. She submitted her article to the British Medical Journal.

Many studies look at the relationship between an exposure and an outcome, hoping to show that a causal relationship exists. The findings may, however, be explained by the existence of a third factor, a confounder.

A confounder has a triangular relationship with both the exposure and the outcome, but most importantly, it is not on the causal pathway (**Figure 8**). It makes it appear as if there is a direct relationship between the exposure and the outcome, or it may even mask an association that would otherwise have been present.

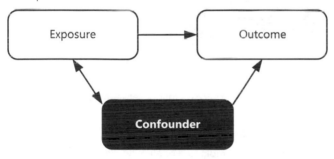

Figure 8 The relationship between the exposure, the outcome and the confounder

To be a confounding factor, the variable must be associated with:

- The exposure but not be the consequence of the exposure
- The outcome, independently of the exposure (ie not an intermediary).

In the example overleaf (**Figure 9**), drinking coffee appears to cause coronary heart disease. Smoking is a confounding factor. It is associated with coffee drinking and it is a risk factor for coronary heart disease, even in people who do not drink coffee.

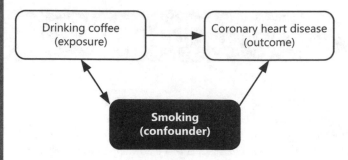

Figure 9 Smoking is a confounding factor

The reverse is not true. Coffee drinking does not confound the relationship between smoking and coronary heart disease, even though it is associated with smoking. Drinking coffee is not a risk factor for coronary heart disease independently of smoking (**Figure 10**).

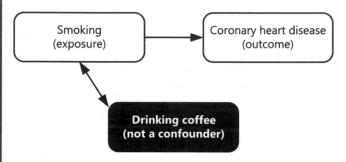

Figure 10 Drinking coffee is not a confounding factor

A **positive confounder** results in an association between two variables that are not associated.

- Example: The association between coffee drinking and lung cancer is positively confounded by smoking. People who drink coffee may also smoke. Smoking is a risk factor for lung cancer even for those people who do not drink coffee.

A **negative confounder** masks an association which is really present.

- Example: The association between poor diet and coronary heart disease may be negatively confounded by exercise. People who exercise regularly may compensate the effects of a poor diet, making it appear that poor diet is not associated with coronary heart disease.

Confounding can cause overestimation or underestimation of the true association and may even change the direction of the observed effect. An example is the confounding by age of an inverse association between level of exercise and heart attacks (younger people taking more rigorous exercise), causing overestimation.

Identification of confounders

Confounding factors differ from bias in that confounding is not usually created by some mistake made by the researchers. Confounding usually arises from a real-life relationship that already exists between the exposures being examined and outcomes under consideration.

Importantly, confounding factors must be identified so that measures can be taken to eliminate them, spread them equally between different arms of the study, or neutralise their effects on the results, using statistical techniques.

Confounders can be measured and controlled for (eg by multiple linear regression) but good study design is essential as one cannot exclude a confounder which was not measured.

Methods to control confounding

At the time of designing the study
- Restriction – certain confounding factors are restricted from entering the sample population using inclusion and exclusion criteria
- Matching – people with confounding factors are allocated equally in the different arms of a study
- Randomisation – confounding factors, known or unknown, can be evenly distributed among the study groups depending on the method of randomisation.

Confounders can exert effects only if they differ between study groups. Restriction or matching may limit the sample size and possible analysis strategies; in particular, one cannot study the effect of a matched variable on an outcome.

At the time of analysis of the study
- Stratification
- Standardisation
- Statistical adjustment.

Stratification

If a potential confounding factor can be identified at the design stage, the data generated during the study can be separated into strata based on that potential confounding factor. This enables the researcher to keep the characteristics of the participants as similar as possible across the study groups (eg age, weight or functional status). Once these strata are identified, separate block randomisation schemes are created for each factor, to ensure that the groups are balanced within each stratum.

Stratification can be achieved by a statistical technique called the Mantel–Haenszel method, which gives adjusted relative risks as a summary measure of the overall risk, or the Mantel–Haenszel estimate of odds ratio, which gives a weighted average of the stratum-specific odds ratios, the weights being dependent upon the numbers of observations in each stratum.

Stratification is unable to control simultaneously for even a moderate number of potential confounders. The number of strata is limited by the sample size needed for each stratum.

Standardisation

The risk in the exposed group is adjusted to that which would have been observed had there been the same confounder distribution as in the unexposed group. For example, if age is a confounding factor, the risk in the exposed group could be adjusted to the age-standardised risk. Standardisation is flexible and reversible. Data collection can be completed before potential confounders are dealt with. However, standardisation becomes difficult when dealing with more than one confounder.

Statistical adjustment using multivariate statistics

This statistical method is used to take confounding factors into account. It analyses the data by using a mathematical model that takes the outcome under consideration as the dependent variable and includes the causal factor and any confounding factors in the equation. These factors are referred to as 'covariables'. The equation allows you to check how much the confounding factors / covariables contribute to the overall effect. When the dependent variables are continuous in nature, multiple linear regression is used. If the variables are binary, logistic regression is used. The advantage of using multivariate analysis is that more than one potential confounder can be considered and the technique is flexible and reversible.

Multivariate statistics can control for a number of confounding factors simultaneously as long as there are at least ten subjects for every variable investigated in a logistic regression situation.

Scenario 6 revisited

Dr Edwards received a letter from the editor of the British Medical Journal. *The editor wrote, "Although a most interesting conclusion, the results of the study are less impressive when confounding variables are considered. Unfortunately, smoking as a confounder has been overlooked. I'm afraid that we cannot consider publishing your study results. I wish you better luck in the future."*

Self-assessment exercise 6

In the following lists of three variables, state which factor, if not identified, would act as a confounding factor in the relationship between the other two variables:

1. Cigarette lighter; smoking cigarettes; lung cancer.

2. Skin cancer; fair skin; blue eyes.

3. Smoking; the oral contraceptive pill, myocardial infarction.

4. Life events; poverty; depression.

TO SUMMARISE, A GOOD STUDY WILL ...
List confounding factors and explain their impact on any relationship under investigation
Describe how confounding factors were controlled at the design and analysis stages

THE PLACEBO EFFECT

Scenario 7

Dr Singh, a rheumatologist, finished writing his first case report. He had seen a patient with arthritis. The patient had visited his general practitioner and had, by the press of a wrong key on the computer, been mistakenly dispensed co-careldopa, a treatment for Parkinson's disease, instead of co-codamol, a pain killer. The patient had unwittingly taken the wrong treatment for a month and, far from experiencing no effect, the patient had dramatically improved pain symptoms. Dr Singh submitted his report to the Lancet, stating that for the first time the pain-killing properties of anti-parkinsonism treatment had been demonstrated, and may lead to a new treatment approach.

Researchers in intervention trials attempt to show whether a treatment improves the health of the subjects. However, subjects may improve simply if they expect to get better with treatment. This effect is so powerful that subjects can improve even if they are unaware that they have been given a placebo, or dummy treatment. A placebo does not have any therapeutic activity for the condition being treated.

The placebo effect

The placebo effect is the name given to the improvement seen in patients when they are in receipt of a placebo treatment. The placebo effect is greater when a patient is given several pills instead of one pill, larger pills instead of smaller pills, and capsules instead of tablets.

One arm in an intervention trial is usually given the active treatment and the other arm is given a placebo treatment. The placebo is used to determine whether any difference in outcome is attributable to the active treatment or to the effect of expectation. If the improvement in the active arm is the same as that in the placebo arm, all the improvement can be attributed to the placebo effect. If the improvement is greater in the active arm, the active treatment is having a beneficial effect over and above that due to the placebo effect.

Placebos

Patients do not enter clinical trials hoping to be allocated to the placebo arm. However, most trials need subjects in the placebo arm. Placebo treatments should be as similar as possible to the active treatment. They should look the same, feel the same, smell the same, taste the same and have the same mode of delivery. A placebo treatment might be sourced from the manufacturer of the active treatment in order to look as similar as possible and only differ in that it has no therapeutic activity. The subject will then be unable to determine whether he/she is in the placebo arm and is more likely to continue in the trial.

It is not always ethical to use a placebo treatment. For example, in some conditions the patient's condition may progress and/or deteriorate if given a placebo. If a beneficial treatment already exists, the new treatment is compared with the standard treatment, not a placebo.

Some organisations argue that all new treatments should be compared in head-to-head trials with the current standard or best treatment, to see if the new treatment is significantly better. However, trials in which an active treatment is not compared with a placebo treatment cannot determine how much of any improvement is due to the placebo effect.

The use of placebos also helps to maintain blinding.

Scenario 7 revisited

The editor of the Lancet wrote back to Dr Singh. He thanked Dr Singh for submitting his case report but noted that, "The placebo effect of co-careldopa needs to be explored and will probably explain the beneficial effects seen. To really demonstrate the efficacy of co-careldopa with pain symptoms, I would suggest a placebo-controlled double-blind strategy is more appropriate. I'll be happy to publish these results if they can be replicated in a better study."

TO SUMMARISE, A GOOD STUDY WILL ...
Explain the role of the placebo effect in any relationship under investigation
Describe any placebo treatment used
Discuss how blinding was maintained when a placebo was used by describing its similarity to the active treatment
Confirm that the study received ethical approval for using a placebo treatment

RESTRICTION

Inclusion criteria and exclusion criteria should normally be listed in the methodology section of a clinical paper.

Inclusion criteria

These criteria determine which people in the target population are eligible to be included in the sample population of a study.

Exclusion criteria

These criteria determine which people in the target population are not eligible to be included in the sample population of a study. Exclusion criteria can be used to eliminate known confounding factors from the study.

In order to minimise selection bias, the inclusion and exclusion criteria must be clearly stated before the study begins. Excessive use of inclusion and exclusion criteria will influence the generalisability of the results, as over-restriction of the sample population will make it unrepresentative of the target population (diagnostic purity bias).

Self-assessment exercise 7

You are developing a study protocol looking at the benefits of the antipsychotic drug, risperidone, in the treatment of schizo-affective disorder in hospital inpatients. Which inclusion and exclusion criteria would you apply?

TO SUMMARISE, A GOOD STUDY WILL ...

List the inclusion criteria and relate them to the aims of the study

List the exclusion criteria and explain the role of confounding factors in any relationship under investigation

Illustrate how many people were included and excluded, often in the form of a table or flowchart

MATCHING

Ideally in a study with more than one arm, the subjects in each arm should be as similar as possible apart from exposure to the risk factor or intervention of interest.

In studies such as case–control and cohort studies, the researchers will recruit the cases first before recruiting a control group. The cases and controls are usually matched, which means that for every case there is a control subject who has similar values of the matching variables. The matching variables are usually demographic characteristics, such as sex, age and ethnicity. The variables are not of interest in themselves.

Matching can also be used to evenly distribute confounding factors. Study participants are chosen to ensure that potential confounding variables are evenly distributed in the two groups being compared. This ensures that any confounding factor that has been identified in the experimental group can also be replicated in the control group.

Matching must be used with caution as it can, like restriction, limit the sample size and possible analysis strategies. It can be difficult to find matching controls, especially with large numbers of matching variables. In these situations, matching may be abandoned in favour of using statistical analyses later to adjust for the variables which would have been matched had there been a sufficient number of controls. This is easier to do in large studies. In small studies, matching is preferred.

TO SUMMARISE, A GOOD STUDY WILL ...

Describe potential confounding factors

Describe how matching was done and any difficulties encountered

Provide a table comparing the baseline demographic and prognostic characteristics of the different groups

RANDOMISATION

This method ensures that all the individuals entering into a study have an equal chance of being allocated to any group within the study. Allocation of participants to specific treatment groups in a random fashion ensures that each group is, on average, as similar as possible to the other group(s).

Randomisation can be divided into three broad areas that all overlap:

- Random number generation
- Randomisation method
- Concealed allocation.

Random number generation

Successful randomisation requires that group assignment cannot be predicted in advance. Some methods of allocation, such as alternate allocation to treatment group or methods based on patient characteristics are not reliably random. These allocation sequences are predictable and not easily concealed, and therefore may reduce the guarantee that allocation has been random, and that no potential participants have been excluded by pre-existing knowledge of the intervention.

Instead, researchers use a variety of techniques to generate a random sequence that can be used to decide allocation:

- Computer random number generation – the most popular method.
- Random number tables – contain a series of numbers which occur equally often and are arranged in a random fashion. Numbers usually have two or more digits
- Shuffled cards or envelopes.

Randomisation methods

Randomisation methods can be divided into:

- **Fixed randomisation:** The randomisation methods are defined and allocation sequences are set up before the start of the trial. Examples include simple randomisation, block randomisation, stratified randomisation and randomised consent.
- **Adaptive randomisation:** The randomised groups are adjusted as the study progresses, to account for imbalances in the numbers in the groups or in response to the outcome data. An example is minimisation.

Fixed randomisation

Simple randomisation

Each subject's allocation is decided at random as each subject enters the study, independently of any other factors. Methods include flipping a coin (for studies with two groups), rolling a dice (for studies with two or more groups) and random number tables and computer-generated random numbers.

With simple randomisation confounding factors, known and unknown, have an equal chance of entering either group but the result may still be unequal group sizes and unequal distribution of confounding factors, particularly in small trials.

Block randomisation

Block randomisation is used to ensure that there are equal numbers of patients in each arm. As subjects are recruited into the sample population, they are not allocated individually as in simple randomisation. Instead, subjects are put into blocks which, when filled, are divided equally into the different arms of the study. The order of this allocation within the block is randomly permuted. Some clinical papers refer to this method as 'permuted block randomisation'.

Stratified randomisation

Simple and block randomisation might not distribute confounding factors equally into the groups. Although the asymmetrical distribution of confounding factors can be dealt with using statistical analyses later, an extension of block randomisation, called 'stratified randomisation', may also help.

In stratified randomisation, subgroups (or stria) containing confounding factors are formed. Within each subgroup, block randomisation takes place. As a result the confounding factor is equally distributed in the different arms.

In small studies it becomes impractical to stratify on more than one or two confounding factors. Minimisation is an alternative method for achieving similarity between study arms.

Other forms of randomisation

Randomised consent method: This is a method used when the study is interested in both the effects of informed consent on treatment efficacy and on the efficacies of the compared treatments.

Quasi-random allocation: A method of allocating subjects to different arms that is not truly random; for example, allocation by date of birth, day of the week, medical record number, month of the year, or the order in which subjects are included in the study (alternation). A quasi-randomised trial uses quasi-random methods of allocating participants to different interventions. There is a greater risk of selection bias in quasi-random trials where allocation is not adequately concealed compared with randomised controlled trials with adequate allocation concealment.

Cluster randomisation: A group of subjects are randomised to the same arm together. The subjects within each unit are called a 'cluster'. In these studies the unit of analysis is the cluster, rather than the individual subjects in that arm. Often a summary statistic for the improvement in each cluster is calculated and compared. Cluster randomisation is most commonly seen in public health and primary care research.

Adaptive randomisation

In adaptive randomisation methods the probability of being allocated to a certain arm in the study is adjusted to maintain similarity between the arms. As an arm becomes imbalanced with subjects of a certain characteristic, the probability of future similar subjects also being allocated to the same arm reduces.

Minimisation is the most commonly used adaptive randomisation method. At the outset, the researchers decide which factors they would like to be present in equal numbers in the different arms. The first subject recruited is allocated to an arm by a random method. Following subjects are allocated to the arm in such a way as to keep all the arms as similar as possible with regard to the predetermined factors. The allocation of each subject therefore depends on the characteristics of the subjects already enrolled. In small studies minimisation is more effective than randomisation in ensuring that the different arms are as similar as possible. Minimisation is also effective when multiple factors need to be distributed evenly.

TO SUMMARISE, A GOOD STUDY WILL ...

Describe how random numbers were generated and by whom

Describe the randomisation method which was employed

Provide a table comparing the baseline demographic and prognostic characteristics of the different groups to show that randomisation was effective

Discuss how concealed allocation was achieved and monitored

CONCEALED ALLOCATION

Scenario 8

Dr Robertson assessed an elderly woman with breathing difficulties and decided she needed hospital treatment. He admitted the woman to a respiratory ward. The ward nurse asked if the patient was eligible for the study he was doing on the efficacy of a new nebuliser treatment. Dr Robertson replied that as the next subject to be recruited was to be allocated to the new treatment arm, he did not think he could risk it with this poorly patient, even though she met the inclusion criteria. He told the ward nurse that the patient would not be taking part in the trial.

The recruitment of subjects into a trial can be adversely affected if the interventions that will be given in each group are known. For example, the ideal result in a treatment study is a significant difference in the outcomes of subjects in the treatment and placebo groups in favour of the new treatment. This difference can be exaggerated by recruiting the 'best' patients to the treatment group and the 'worst' patients to the placebo group.

Even if randomisation is employed to allocate patients to groups, this problem may still arise as the randomisation schedule is often published in advance. If it is known that the next individual will be allocated to the new treatment group according to the randomisation schedule, an individual who may not do so well may be overlooked for recruitment into the study. Instead, the researcher may wait for someone who will do very well in the new treatment group.

Concealed allocation

Concealment means the interventions in the different arms of the study are kept secret. As a result, the researchers are unaware of the intervention in the group to which a subject will be allocated, should that individual agree to be in the study. This avoids both conscious and unconscious selection of patients into the study. 'Concealed allocation' is a vital part of the randomisation process.

A good study will not have the same people recruiting and randomising subjects.

There are a number of ways in which concealed allocation can be achieved. For example, with a centralised concealment scheme in a multicentre trial, the clinician checks for eligibility, gains consent, decides on whether to enrol patients, and then calls the randomisation service to obtain the treatment allocation. This communication can happen by telephone or electronically on the internet.

In situations in which remote randomisation may not be feasible, a set of tamper-evident envelopes that look identical may be provided to each site. The envelopes are opaque and well sealed, and the sequence of opening the envelopes is monitored regularly. Other techniques include using coded containers in which treatments from numbered bottles that appear otherwise identical are administered sequentially.

Concealed allocation and blinding

The two terms are often confused because they both involve keeping interventions secret. Concealed allocation is part of the randomisation and allocation procedures. It seeks to eliminate selection bias. Blinding happens after randomisation and aims to reduce observation bias.

Scenario 8 revisited

Dr Robertson's study concluded that the new nebuliser treatment was of major benefit to patients with breathing difficulties and it would save lives if it was given as a first-line treatment. He presented his findings at the hospital's academic meeting. In the audience was the ward nurse. At the end of the presentation, after Dr Robertson invited questions and comments, she said, "As you were aware of the treatments being given in each group and the allocation sequence, your selection of patients was biased and ended up widening the difference between the groups. Does selection bias not make your results invalid?"

TO SUMMARISE, A GOOD STUDY WILL ...

Include concealed allocation as part of the randomisation process
Describe the people involved in recruiting and allocating subjects
Discuss how concealed allocation was achieved and monitored

Scenario 9

Dr Joseph analysed the results of a trial on the usefulness of psychological interventions in patients suffering chronic pain. In one arm of the study, the patients received 20 weekly sessions with a psychologist, exploring their perceptions of pain. In the control arm, the patients were invited to chat to a nurse about their daily routine. The psychologists dramatically reduced pain scores compared with the 'placebo' intervention. Dr Joseph wrote to his Hospital Board, suggesting that sessions with psychologists were a cost-effective intervention for his patients and could reduce the need for pain clinic appointments.

Scenario 10

Dr Webb was amazed by the results of her trial investigating a new mood-stabilising medication for patients suffering with bipolar disorder. Compared with patients taking lithium, the patients taking the new treatment reported fewer symptoms and they were pleased they did not need regular blood tests to monitor drug levels. She submitted her results to the British Journal of Psychiatry and recommended that lithium was no longer the gold standard treatment for bipolar patients. She hoped that her results would be the topic of the journal's editorial.

The behaviour of researchers and study participants can be influenced by what they know or believe. If participants in a trial are aware they are receiving a placebo or active intervention, the answers they give may be influenced by this knowledge. Similarly, the researchers may also be influenced by any awareness of which individuals are receiving the different interventions. The behaviour of study participants and researchers can lead to bias, as the subjective answers and assessments might not actually mirror the truth. This bias often occurs at a subconscious level.

Blinding, sometimes called 'masking', overcomes this problem. Treatment is termed 'blind' when the subject and/or researcher do not know what trial treatments are being administered.

- **Open trial:** No blinding is used.
- **Single blinding:** Either the researcher or the subject is blind to the allocation.
- **Double blinding:** The researcher and the subject are not aware of the treatment being administered. The interventions should appear identical for each treatment group.

- **Triple blinding:** Knowledge of the treatment is concealed from the researcher, subject and the analyst processing the results.

Blind assessment is used to describe the assessment of the outcome measures during and at the end of the study without knowledge of what the treatment groups are. Blind assessment by a third party is useful in open trials, case–control studies and cohort studies.

The blinding procedure should be clearly stated in the methodology section of the study. As a result of blinding, the groups in the trial should be treated equally.

The use of placebos helps to maintain blinding. If the interventions are very different, a **double-dummy** technique may be used, in which all the subjects appear to receive both interventions, although one is a placebo, in order to maintain blinding.

Although desirable, blinding is not always possible. Open trials or single-blind studies are often employed when investigating invasive or psychological interventions.

Scenario 9 revisited
The Medical Director of the hospital wrote back to Dr Joseph, stating, "It is hardly surprising that the psychotherapy patients got better. They were aware they were getting the new intervention. While I accept that talking therapies are hard to blind, we must not rush into making costly decisions based on such trials."

Scenario 10 revisited
Unfortunately the research article was rejected by the peer review process. The Editor of the British Journal of Psychiatry wrote to Dr Webb, "Unfortunately, blinding in your study was compromised because the patients taking lithium had regular blood tests. It was surely obvious who was taking lithium and who was tak-ing the new mood-stabiliser drug. To maintain blinding and eliminate observation bias, everyone should have had the same blood tests. Sham results should have been reported for patients not taking lithium. This major oversight means I cannot publish your article. I hope this news is not too depressing for you."

TO SUMMARISE, A GOOD STUDY WILL ...

Describe how blinding was implemented

Discuss the use of placebos and other sham interventions in helping to maintain blinding

Figure 11 The study pathway

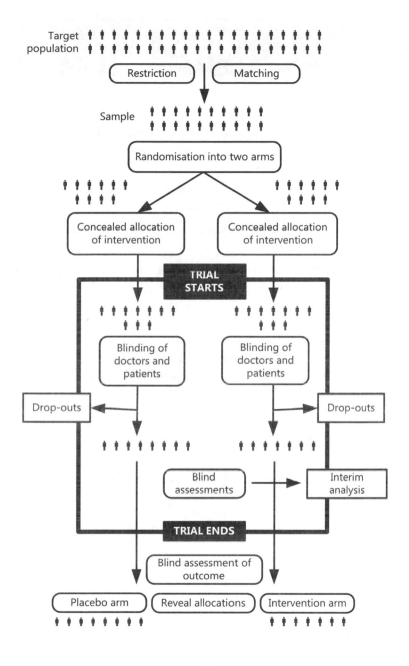

ENDPOINTS

Studies report results in terms of the endpoints that were measured. There are numerous endpoints that can be used in studies, for example mortality, disease progression, disability, improvement of symptoms in patients and quality of life measures.

Ideally, changes in endpoints should help doctors make better decisions for their patients and have some clinical significance.

There are three main types of endpoint to consider when assessing the outcomes of a study.

Clinical endpoint: A measurement of a direct clinical outcome, such as mortality, morbidity or survival.

Surrogate endpoint: A measurement of an outcome used as a substitute for a clinically meaningful endpoint. The surrogate endpoint must fully capture the net effect of the intervention on the clinical endpoint. Although surrogate endpoints are believed to be predictive of important clinical outcomes, the relationship is not guaranteed. They are used because they allow effects to be measured sooner. For example, blood pressure reduction may be used as a surrogate endpoint because blood pressure is a risk factor for cerebrovascular and cardiovascular events; for atherosclerosis, cardiovascular mortality or myocardial infarction, angiography or ultrasound imaging can be used.

Surrogate markers are also used in phases 1 and 2 of clinical trials – that is, the early stages of drug development. They may also be used in phase 3 trials, but there is then careful consideration of how accurately the surrogate marker reflects the clinical outcome in question and whether it will be accurate and reliable. Sample sizes for studies using surrogate markers can be smaller and the trial does not have to be as long-lasting, because changes in the surrogate endpoints usually occur before the clinical event occurs.

Composite endpoint: These combine several measurements into a single composite endpoint, using a pre-specified algorithm. This is useful when any one event occurs too infrequently to be an endpoint and overcomes the problem of insufficient power in a study. The **primary endpoint** – that is, the health parameter that is measured in all study participants to detect a response to treatment – must be specified. Conclusions about the effectiveness of treatment should focus on this measurement. **Secondary endpoints** are other parameters that are measured in all study participants to help describe the effect of treatment. Ideally all the composite endpoints should be of similar importance to the patient and occur with similar frequency.

Measuring endpoints – validity and reliability

As well as specifying which endpoints were used, a study should describe how these endpoints were measured or detected. Clinical endpoints tend to be objective and easily measured, eg the patient died or the patient lived or was cured. Surrogate endpoints are more widely used but are more prone to subjective assessments and differences of opinion. Problems can arise if the measurements are not made consistently.

Researchers use measuring techniques and instruments that have been shown to be valid and reliable. **Validity** refers to the extent to which a test measures what it is supposed to measure. **Reliability** refers to how consistent a test is on repeated measurements.

The meaning of these two terms can be clarified by making an analogy with target practice (**Figure 12**). Hitting the bulls-eye on the target is 'validity' or correctness. Repeatedly hitting the same point is 'reliability' or consistency.

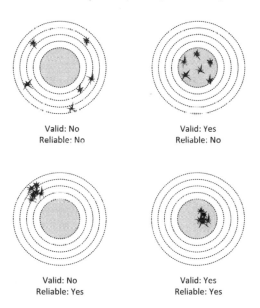

Valid: No
Reliable: No

Valid: Yes
Reliable: No

Valid: No
Reliable: Yes

Valid: Yes
Reliable: Yes

Figure 12 The relationship between validity and reliability

TO SUMMARISE, A GOOD STUDY WILL ...

Clearly state the endpoint of interest
Relate the endpoint to the clinical question
Describe how the endpoint was detected and measured

VALIDITY

Scenario 11

Dr Harrison looked at the next research proposal submitted for ethics approval. A junior doctor wished to compare the efficacy of a new thyroxine depot injection against that of thyroxine tablets, in young men with hypothyroidism. She proposed a cohort study assessing the severity of symptoms by the television viewing time of each subject at home, as hypothyroid patients tended to be tired all the time. She hypothesised that thyroxine treatment would improve hypothyroid symptoms, marked by a reduction in the amount of television viewed.

The term '**validity**' refers to the extent to which a test measures what it is supposed to measure. There are many subtypes of validity.

Criterion validity

This is made up of predictive, concurrent, convergent and discriminant validity. It is used to demonstrate the accuracy of a measure or procedure by comparing it with another measure or procedure that has been demonstrated to be valid.

Predictive validity: The extent to which the test is able to predict something it should theoretically be able to predict. For example, a written examination would have predictive validity if it measured performance in high school and successfully predicted employment status in adulthood.

Concurrent validity: The extent to which the test is able to distinguish between groups it should theoretically be able to distinguish between. For example, a questionnaire would have concurrent validity if it successfully distinguished sufferers of chest pain due to angina from sufferers of chest pain due to gastritis.

Convergent validity: The extent to which the test is similar to other tests that it theoretically should be similar to. For example, a digital thermometer would have convergent validity with a mercury-based thermometer if it returned similar results.

Discriminant validity: The extent to which the test is not similar to other tests that it theoretically should not be similar to. For example, a postgraduate assessment of critical appraisal skills of doctors would have discriminant validity if it returned results dissimilar to a multiple-choice question paper testing knowledge of diseases.

Other types of validity

Face validity: The extent to which the test, on superficial consideration, measures what it is supposed to measure. For example, a test measuring the exercise tolerance of patients and relating it to respiratory disease severity would have face validity.

Content validity: The extent to which the test measures variables that are related to that which should be measured by the test. For example, a questionnaire assessing angina severity would have content validity if the questions centred on the ability to do everyday tasks that made the heart work harder.

Construct validity: The extent to which the test measures a theoretical concept by a specific measuring device or procedure. For example, an IQ test would have construct validity if its results reflected the theoretical concept of intelligence.

Incremental validity: The extent to which the test provides a significant improvement in addition to the use of another approach. A test has incremental validity if it helps more than not using it. For example, ultrasound scanning gives better estimates of fetal gestation age than clinical examination alone.

Scenario 11 revisited

Dr Harrison wrote back to the young researcher, stating that, "Selecting patients and assessing them on the basis of their viewing habits seems inappropriate to me. Hypothyroid patients may do many things apart from increase their television viewing time (and I'm not even sure about that!), so it appears to me that a more valid assessment method is required."

TO SUMMARISE, A GOOD STUDY WILL ...

Describe what was measured and how this related to the endpoints

RELIABILITY

Scenario 12

Dr Nolan was supervising a class of first-year medical students. All the students were asked to take each other's blood pressure until they were comfortable using a sphygmomanometer. Dr Nolan noticed that, halfway through the session, some of the students looked bemused. He asked one student what the matter was. "It's these sphygmomanometers," said the student, "they never give the same result twice!" After the session, Dr Nolan wrote to the Clinical Tutor, suggesting that an investment be made in better equipment.

Many studies involve the measurement of one or more variables. Good research technique involves commenting on the reliability of these measurements – that is, the consistency of test results on repeat measurements. Repeat measurements can be by the same person, by more than one person, and/or across time. Good reliability ensures consistency of the results and conclusions that are being drawn from the study.

Test–retest reliability: Refers to the level of agreement between the initial test results and the results of repeat measurements made at a later date.

Inter-rater reliability: Refers to the level of agreement between assessments made by two or more raters at the same time. This measure of agreement can be quantified as a correlation coefficient, the kappa (Cohen's) statistic (κ). Kappa is also known as the 'chance-corrected proportional agreement statistic'.

Measurements can agree purely by chance. The kappa statistic (κ) indicates the level of the agreement between measurements by different raters and gives an indication as to whether this agreement is more than can be expected by chance. If agreement is no more than expected by chance, then $\kappa = 0$. With perfect agreement, $\kappa = 1$ (**Table 9**). To avoid low kappa values, measurements by researchers can be improved by simply agreeing criteria and measurement conditions. One disadvantage of this measurement of agreement is that it is sensitive to the prevalence / proportion of individuals in each group.

To calculate kappa:

$$\text{kappa} = (P_O - P_E)/(1 - P_E)$$

P_O = observed agreement

P_E = agreement expected by chance

KAPPA	STRENGTH OF AGREEMENT
0	Chance agreement only
<0.2	Poor agreement beyond chance
0.21–0.4	Fair agreement beyond chance
0.41–0.6	Moderate agreement beyond chance
0.61–0.8	Good agreement beyond chance
0.81 – 1.0	Very good agreement beyond chance
1.0	Perfect agreement

Table 9 Kappa (κ) and the strength of agreement

Kappa is for use with tests measuring categorical variables. For nominal ordered data, kappa is preferably weighted (κ_w) to allow for any near misses.

Cronbach's α: This is used with complicated tests with several parts or for measuring several variables. If Cronbach's α is ≥0.5 there is moderate agreement and if ≥0.8 there is excellent agreement.

Intra-class correlation coefficient: This is for use with tests measuring quantitative variables. It describes the extent to which two continuous measures taken by different people, or two measurements taken by the same person on different occasions, are related.

Other types of reliability include:

Intra-rater reliability: This looks at the level of agreement between assessments by one rater of the same material at two or more different times.

Alternative-form reliability: This describes reliability of similar forms of the test, looking at the same material either at the same time or immediately consecutively. For example, the temperature reading from a mercury thermometer could be compared with that from a digital thermometer.

Split-half reliability: This describes the reliability of a test that is divided in two, with each half being used to assess the same material under similar circumstances.

Scenario 12 revisited

The Clinical Tutor wrote back to Dr Nolan, thanking him for his feedback. He went on, "The issue of reliability is indeed an important one in blood pressure measurements. I don't think simply having a new set of sphygmomanometers will make much of a difference, because the reliability of the measure is never going to be perfect, no matter who uses the sphygmomanometer!"

TO SUMMARISE, A GOOD STUDY WILL ...

Provide evidence that measuring instruments are reliable, usually by referring to earlier studies

Quote correlation coefficient values

Describe how reliability was improved by training and standardisation

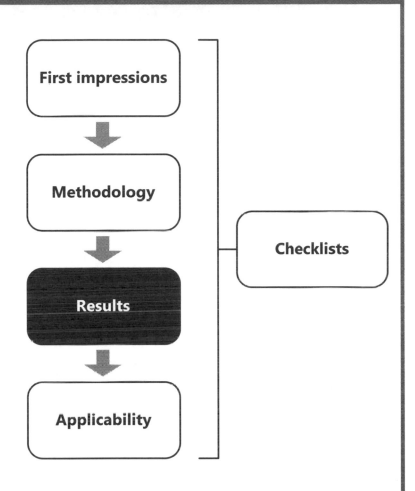

TYPES OF DATA

Data can be classified as either qualitative or quantitative.

Qualitative data

Qualitative data are also known as categorical or non-numerical data.

Examples of qualitative data:

- Single, engaged, married, divorced, widowed
- Poor, average, good, excellent
- Red, yellow, blue, silver, green
- Cured, not cured.

Quantitative data

Quantitative data are also known as numerical data and are classified as either discrete or continuous.

Discrete data have a finite number of possible values and tend to be made up of integers (or whole numbers). Counts are examples of discrete data:

- Number of pupils absent each day from school: 7, 3, 13, 14, 4, 2
- Waiting time to see a doctor in days: 2, 1, 3, 2, 1, 2, 1.

Continuous data have infinite possibilities. Continuous data values can include decimal places.

- Diameter of tumours: 1.23 cm, 1.78 cm, 2.25 cm,
- Weight of patients: 67.234 kg, 89.935 kg, 101.563 kg

Quantitative data can be converted into categorical data by using cut-off points (**Table 10**). Results of rating scales are often converted into cured/not-cured categories. This is because categorical data are easier to tabulate and analyse.

BLOOD PRESSURE (QUANTITATIVE DATA)		BLOOD PRESSURE (CATEGORIES)
80/30 mmHg		Hypotensive
120/70 mmHg		Normotensive
145/85 mmHg		Normotensive
160/85 mmHg		Normotensive
150/100 mmHg		Hypertensive
165/105 mmHg		Hypertensive

Table 10 Converting quantitative data to categorical data

Measuring instruments and data collection

The measuring instrument used to measure data will determine the type of data collected, for example:

- Fun weighing machine – results given as skinny, normal, fat, too fat! (qualitative data)
- Digital weighing machine – results given in kg to two decimal places (quantitative continuous data).

MEASURING DATA

Measuring data involves using one of four different types of scales. Qualitative data tend to be measured on nominal or ordinal scales. Quantitative data tend to be measured on interval or ratio scales.

Nominal scales

A nominal scale is organised in categories which have no inherent order and which bear no mathematical relationship to each other. Nominal data can be subdivided into binary or multi-category data:

- **Binary (or dichotomous) data:** There are two mutually exclusive categories. Examples include dead or alive, improved or not improved, male or female.
- **Multi-category data:** There are three or more categories. An example is marital status – single, engaged, married, divorced. Another example is hair colour – blond, brunette, brown, black, ginger.

Ordinal scales

An ordinal scale is organised in categories that have an inherent order or rank. The categories are not quantified, so the interval between categories is not meaningful, for example.

- Social classes: I, II, III, IV, V
- Severity of disease: mild, moderate, severe.

Interval scales

An interval scale is organised in a meaningful way, with the differences between points being equal across the scale. Interval data have no true starting point. The value zero on an interval scale has no special meaning. An example is:

- Celsius temperature scale.

Ratio scales

A ratio scale is the same as an interval scale but there is a true zero, eg:

- Kelvin temperature scale.

Self-assessment exercise 8

1. What is the data type for each of the variables below?
   a. The diagnosis of patients on a ward
   b. The sex of patients
   c. The weight of patients
   d. The staging of cancer
   e. The age of patients
   f. The ethnicity of patients
   g. The blood cholesterol level
   h. Patient blood groups
   i. Body temperature
   j. Marital status
   k. Education level

DESCRIBING DATA FROM ONE SAMPLE

Once data have been collected, they need to be summarised in some way. The description of a single set of data should include an indication of the **central tendency** of the data set and a measure of the **spread** of the data around this central tendency. The choice of statistical tests to describe a single set of data depends on the type of data collected.

Categorical data (mode, frequency)

Mode: The most common value.

Frequency: The number of values in each category.

For example, from Table 10:

- the mode is 'normotensive'
- the frequency is:
    - hypotensive (1 observation)
    - normotensive (3 observations)
    - hypertensive (2 observations).

Non-normally distributed data (median, range, interquartile range)

As shown in **Figure 13**, in non-normally distributed data, the data values are distributed asymmetrically across the distribution.

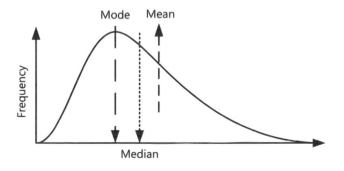

Figure 13 A non-normally distributed data set (positively skewed)

Median: From the Latin for 'middle', the median represents the middle value of ordered data observations. With an even number of data values, the median is the average of the two values that lie on either side of the middle place (**Table 11**).

The advantage of the median estimation is that it is robust to outliers; that is, it is not affected by aberrant points (unlike the mean). This could also be considered a disadvantage as the value of the median gives no indication about the existence of extreme outlying values.

Range: This is the difference between the lowest and highest values in the data set. It is useful for skewed data but it is not robust to aberrant values.

DATA SET	MEDIAN	RANGE
1, 2, 3, 3, 5	3	5 − 1 = 4
1, 2, 3, 3, 5, 7, 8, 10	(3+5 / 2) = 4	10 − 1 = 9

Table 11 Example calculations of median and range

Interquartile range (IQR): This is a 'mini' range because it focuses on the spread of the middle 50% of the data. It is usually reported alongside the median value of the data set.

The data are ranked in order and divided into four equal parts (irrespective of their values). The points at 25%, 50% and 75% of the distribution are identified. These are known as the quartiles and the median is the second quartile. The interquartile range is between the first and third quartiles (**Figure 14**).

Unlike the range, the interquartile range is not influenced by outliers and is relatively easy to calculate. However, the interquartile range does not incorporate all the presented values.

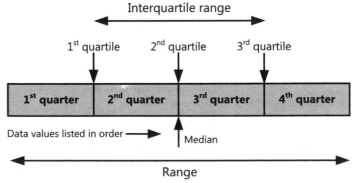

Figure 14 Comparing the range and the interquartile range

If the number of data values is not divisible by four, first identify the median value and then calculate the first and third quartiles by the middle values between the median and the end of the ranges.

Normally distributed data (mean, standard deviation)

A normal distribution, also known as a 'Gaussian distribution', is a perfectly symmetric bell-shaped curve, as shown in (**Figure 15**).

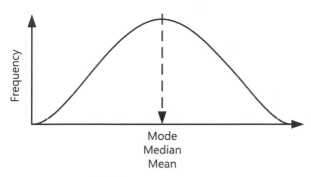

Figure 15 Normal distribution

Mean: The sum of all the values divided by the number of values:

$$mean = \frac{sum\ of\ all\ the\ values}{the\ number\ of\ values}$$

$$\overline{x} = \frac{\Sigma x}{n}$$

The mean uses all the data and is easy to calculate; however, it is still not robust to aberrant values and can be difficult to interpret.

In a perfect normal distribution, the mean, median and mode are of equal value and lie in the centre of the distribution.

Standard deviation (SD): A statistical measure that describes the degree of data spread about the mean – the amount the values will deviate from the mean.

Standard deviation is calculated as the square root of the variance. The variance is the sum of all the differences between all the values and the mean, squared, and divided by the total number of observations minus 1 (the degrees of freedom).

$$standard\ deviation = \sqrt{v} = \sqrt{\frac{\Sigma (x - \overline{x})^2}{n - 1}}$$

The extent of the bell shape in a normal distribution is dependent upon the standard deviation. A key property of the normal distribution is that we can calculate the proportion of the observations that will lie between any two values of the variable as long as we know the mean and standard deviation.

If observations follow a normal distribution, the standard deviation is a useful measure of the spread of these observations:

- A range covered by 1 SD above the mean and 1 SD below the mean includes 68% of the observations (ie the area under the curve) (**Figure 16**).

- A range of 2 SDs (1.96) above and below the mean includes 95% of the observations.

- A range of 3 SDs (2.58) above and below the mean includes 99.7% of the observations.

The larger the standard deviation, the greater the spread of observations around the mean.

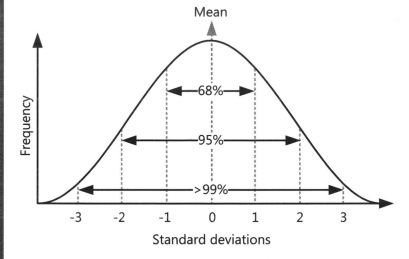

Figure 16 1, 2 and 3 standard deviations shown on a normal distribution

z score: Converts the value of an observation into the number of standard deviations that observation lies from the mean of the distribution. A z score is calculated by subtracting the mean from the observation and dividing the difference by the standard deviation.

So far, we have discussed the normal distribution curve. Two other distributions to consider are **binomial** and **Poisson** distributions, which can be used for discrete random variables.

Measures of shape

The **coefficient of skewness** is a measure of symmetry.

Negatively skewed distribution: The distribution has an extended tail to the left and has a negative coefficient of skewness.

Positively skewed distribution: The distribution has an extended tail to the right and has a positive coefficient of skewness.

Symmetric distribution: This has a coefficient of skewness of zero.

Coefficient of kurtosis: This measures the peakedness of a distribution.

Self-assessment exercise 9

1. In this data set: 1, 2, 2, 3, 3, 3, 4, 4, 5
   a. What is the mode?
   b. What are frequencies?
   c. What is the median?
   d. What is the range?
   e. What is the mean?

2. In this data set: 5, 10, 15, 20, 100
   a. What is the median?
   b. What is the range?
   c. What is the mean?
   d. Which describes the central tendency of this data set better
      – the median or the mean?

3. In this data set: 5, 10, 15, 20, 25, 30, 35, 40, 45, 50, 60, 70
   a. What is the median?
   b. What is the range?
   c. What is the interquartile range?

4. In this data set: 3, 13, 44, 45, 51, 56, 66, 75, 91, 102
   a. What is the mean?
   b. What is the standard deviation?
   c. What is the range in which 95% of observations will lie?

INFERRING POPULATION RESULTS FROM SAMPLES

To generalise the result from a random sample to the target population, two concepts need to be understood:

- Standard error
- Confidence intervals

Standard error (SE)

Suppose that an experiment is set up to measure the mean height of the population. A random sample of the population will be selected to take part in the study. The results from the sample will be generalised to the population.

If the study is repeated with a new random sample, the mean height from this new sample may not be the same as that from the first random sample. Indeed, repeating the study several times may produce a series of different mean heights. This is shown in **Table 12**.

	MEAN HEIGHT	STANDARD DEVIATION
Sample 1	1.65	0.12
Sample 2	1.58	0.23
Sample 3	1.63	0.19
Sample 4	1.88	0.22
Sample 5	1.59	0.18
Sample 6	1.44	0.20
Sample 7	1.63	0.05
Sample 8	1.49	0.14

Table 12 Mean heights (in metres) and standard deviations from different samples

If these sample means are themselves plotted on a graph, they too will follow a normal distribution with their own mean and standard deviation (**Figure 17**). The standard deviation of the sample means has its own name: **standard error**.

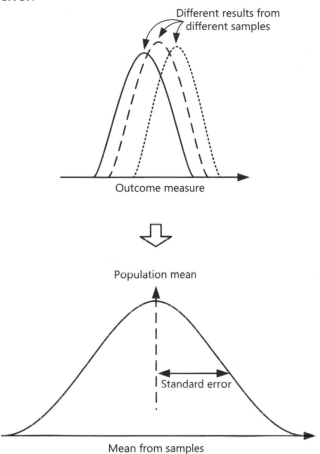

Figure 17 Population mean and standard error

standard error of a sample of sample size $n = \dfrac{standard\ deviation}{\sqrt{n}}$

n = number of observations in the sample

The more observations you have, the smaller will be the standard error – that is, the more likely the sample mean ($\bar{x}$) reflects the true mean value (μ) of a parameter in the general population.

Confidence intervals

Suppose we want to know the mean height of 500 pupils attending a school.

- If all 500 pupils are in our sample, we are 100% confident that we will calculate the correct mean height from all the height measurements we take.

- If our sample is 499 pupils, we are still very confident that the mean height we calculate from our sample will be very similar to the mean height of the target population. The mean height for all 500 pupils may be a bit higher or a bit lower, but the difference if it exists will be very small indeed.

- If our sample is 400 pupils, we are slightly less confident that the mean value we calculate lies close to the real mean value for all the pupils. If we had to guess where the real value lies, we would quote a small range either side of the value we have calculated.

- If our sample is only 50 pupils, we would be even less confident in our result. Even if the result is correct, we don't know it is, so we are less confident. The range in which we think the true value lies will be wider.

Confidence intervals measure the uncertainty in measurements. They can be described as a range of values which, when quoted in relation to an estimate, express the degree of uncertainty around that estimate.

The width of the confidence interval indicates the precision of the estimate. The 95% confidence interval is routinely quoted – it is the range within which we can be 95% confident that the true value for the population lies.

For example, for a mean height of 1.25 m with a 95% confidence interval (95% CI) of 1.1 m and 1.4 m, we are 95% confident that the true mean height value lies between 1.1 m and 1.4 m.

We can make a wide estimate with a high degree of confidence or a more precise estimate with a lower degree of confidence. The larger the sample, the less variable the observations are, the more likely the results are to be true – that is, the narrower the confidence interval and the more confidence one can have in making inferences about the population parameters.

> 95% confidence interval for a population mean =
> mean ± 1.96 × standard error

- When quoted alongside a difference between two groups (eg mean difference), a confidence interval that includes 0 is statistically non-significant.

- When quoted alongside a ratio (eg relative risk, odds ratio), a confidence interval that includes 1 is statistically non-significant.

Self-assessment exercise 10

1. In this data set: 10, 12, 15, 17, 18, 19, 21
    a. What is the mean?
    b. What is the median?
    c. What is the standard deviation?
    d. What is the standard error?

2. In this data set: 10, 12, 15, 17, 18, 19, 91
    a. What is the mean?
    b. What is the median?
    c. What is the standard deviation?
    d. What is the standard error?

EPIDEMIOLOGICAL DATA

Epidemiology is the scientific study of the distribution, causes and control of diseases in populations. Studies frequently provide epidemiological data to describe the disease or population of interest.

There are two main measures of disease frequency: **incidence** and **prevalence**.

Incidence

Incidence: The rate of occurrence of new cases over a period of time in a defined population (**Figure 18**). It is a measure of the risk of disease.

$$incidence = \frac{\text{number of new cases over a period of time}}{\text{population size}}$$

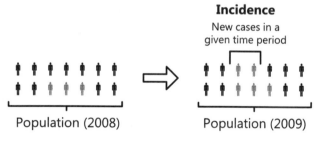

Incidence

New cases in a given time period

Population (2008)   Population (2009)

Figure 18 Incidence

The incidence can be given as a **crude rate**, which is the rate that applies to the whole population without any adjustment. A **specific rate** may be given which only applies to a subgroup in the population.

Mortality rate: This is a type of incidence rate that expresses the risk of death over a period of time in a population.

$$mortality\ rate = \frac{\text{number of deaths over a period of time}}{\text{population size}}$$

- **Standardised mortality rate:** The mortality rate is adjusted to compensate for a confounder, for example age.

- **Standardised mortality ratio:** The ratio of the observed standardised mortality rate (from the study population) to the expected standardised mortality rate (from the standard population). The reference value is 100. Converting a mortality rate into a ratio makes it easier to compare different populations. The lower the ratio, the better.

- **Hospital standardised mortality ratio (HSMR):** A measure of overall mortality in hospitals, used in conjunction with other indicators to assess quality of care. HSMR is adjusted for many factors, including sex, age, socioeconomic deprivation, diagnosis and method of patient admission to hospital.

In 2009 a report by the Healthcare Commission detailed a catalogue of failings at Mid Staffordshire NHS Foundation Trust which were only uncovered when unusually high mortality rates at the hospital triggered alerts[1]. The HSMR for the hospital for 2005/06 was 127, meaning that 27% more patients died than might be expected. It was estimated that between 2005 and 2008, 400 more people died at the hospital than would be expected. The Chairman of the Trust resigned, the Chief Executive was suspended and an independent inquiry was launched.

1   Investigation into Mid Staffordshire NHS Foundation Trust: Commission for Healthcare Audit and Inspection, March 2009 ISBN 978-1-84562-220-6

Morbidity rate: This is the rate of occurrence of new non-fatal cases of the disease in a defined population at risk over a given time period.

$$\text{morbidity rate} = \frac{\text{number of new non-fatal cases over a period of time}}{\text{size of population at risk}}$$

- **Standardised morbidity rate:** The morbidity rate is adjusted to compensate for a confounder.

- **Standardised morbidity ratio:** Ratio of the observed standardised morbidity rate (from the study population) to the expected standardised morbidity rate (from the standard population).

Prevalence

Point prevalence: The proportion of a defined population having the disease at a given point in time (**Figure 19**). Prevalence is useful for planning health services.

$$\text{point prevalence} = \frac{\text{number of people with the disease at a given time}}{\text{size of population at the same time}}$$

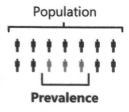

Figure 19 Prevalence

Incidence and prevalence are related by the following equation:

prevalence at any time point = incidence × average duration of the disease

Period prevalence: The proportion of a population that has the disease

$$\text{period prevalence} = \frac{\text{number of people with the disease or developing the disease in a period of time}}{\text{size of population at the same time}}$$

during a given time period (such as annual prevalence).

Lifetime prevalence: This is the proportion of a population that either has or has had the disease at a given point in time.

Self-assessment exercise 11

1. A cohort study was carried out on 200 men. Half of the participants had been exposed to passive smoking while working in pubs. The other half of the participants had not been exposed to passive smoking. After 10 years, there were four cases of lung cancer in the exposed group and one case in the unexposed group. What is the annual incidence rate of lung cancer in the exposed group? What is the annual incidence rate in the unexposed group? What is the overall annual incidence rate?

2. The incidence of cystic fibrosis is 1 in 2500 births. How many new cases will a paediatrician expect to see over ten years if the hospital she works in delivers 90 babies a month?

3. The annual mortality rate for acute pancreatitis is 1.3 per 100 000. If there are 60 million people in the United Kingdom, how many deaths from acute pancreatitis are expected every week?

4. 85 000 people in the United Kingdom have multiple sclerosis. What is the prevalence rate per 100 000 of the population if the United Kingdom population is 60 million people?

5. What will happen to the prevalence of a disease if there is:
   a. Immigration of cases into the area?
   b. Emigration of cases out of the area?
   c. Immigration of healthy persons into the area?
   d. An increase in the case fatality rate?

RISKS AND ODDS

Describing risk in a group

Risk and odds apply to a single group of people.

Risk: In clinical research, risk has the same meaning as probability. Risk is the probability of something happening. Risk is the number of times an event is likely to occur divided by the total number of events possible. It is expressed as P and is presented either as a number between 0 and 1 or as a percentage.

Odds: Odds is also another way of expressing chance. The odds is the ratio of the number of times an event is likely to occur divided by the number of times it is likely not to occur. This is expressed as a ratio or fraction.

For example, if someone is expecting a baby:

the risk of it being a girl is 1/2, or 50%

the odds of it being a girl is $1/1 = 1$ – that is, it is as likely to be a girl as it is not to be a girl.

Comparing risk between groups

If two groups are being compared, relative risk and odds ratio compare the two groups with respect to the likelihood of an event occurring, and describe the risk of subjects having an outcome in the presence of an exposure.

2 × 2 contingency tables

The most common way to calculate the risk ratio is to start by tabulating the results in a **contingency table**, also known as **2 × 2 table (Table 13)**. The contingency table consists of rows and columns of cells. The frequencies of the events are recorded in the relevant boxes.

Contingency tables can be a source of confusion, because there are different ways of displaying the same information. Always maintain a consistent approach by having the exposure factor or intervention across the rows and the disease status or outcome status down the columns. Disease status positive is always the worst outcome, such as death.

		OUTCOME STATUS		
		positive	negative	Totals
EXPOSURE	positive	a	b	a + b
	negative	c	d	c + d
Totals		a + c	b + d	a + b + c + d

Table 13 2 × 2 contingency table

Other aspects of risk can be derived from the 2 × 2 contingency table (**Table 14**).

	FORMULA
Control event rate (CER) (outcome event rate in control group)	$\dfrac{c}{c + d}$
Experimental event rate (EER) (outcome event rate in experimental group)	$\dfrac{a}{a + b}$
Absolute risk reduction (ARR)	$CER - EER$
Relative risk (RR)	$\dfrac{EER}{CER}$
Relative risk reduction (RRR)	$\dfrac{CER - EER}{CER}$
Numbers needed to treat (NNT)	$\dfrac{1}{ARR}$
Odds of outcome in exposed group	$\dfrac{a}{b}$
Odds of outcome in non-exposed group	$\dfrac{c}{d}$
Odds ratio	$\dfrac{a/b}{c/d} = \dfrac{ad}{bc}$

Table 14 Derivation of other aspects of risk from the 2 × 2 contingency table

Absolute risk

The incidence rate of the outcome in the group (which can be the treated or the untreated population).

$$\text{Control event rate (CER)} = \text{risk in subjects not exposed} = \frac{c}{c + d}$$

$$\text{Experimental event rate (EER)} = \text{risk in subjects exposed} = \frac{a}{a + b}$$

Absolute risk reduction

Absolute risk reduction (ARR) is the absolute risk in the control group minus the absolute risk in the experimental group:

$$\text{Absolute risk reduction} = CER - EER$$

Relative risk

Relative risk (RR) or risk ratio is the absolute risk in the experimental group divided by the absolute risk in the control group:

$$\text{Relative risk} = \frac{EER}{CER}$$

- If the relative risk is statistically significantly different from 1, there is evidence of an **association**.
- If the relative risk is equal to 1, there is **no risk difference** between the groups.
- If the relative risk is greater than 1, there is **an increased risk** among those exposed to the factor.
- If the relative risk is less than 1, the factor is **protective** against the disease.

Relative risk reduction

Relative risk reduction (RRR) is the proportional reduction in rates of outcomes between experimental and control subjects in a study.

$$\text{Relative risk reduction} = \frac{CER - EER}{CER}$$

Number needed to treat

The number needed to treat (NNT) is the number of subjects that must be treated with the intervention, compared with the control, for one extra subject to experience the beneficial effect. It is the reciprocal of the absolute risk reduction between two interventions. The lower the value of NNT, the better. The minimum value for NNT is 1; the maximum value is infinity.

$$\text{Number needed to treat} = \frac{1}{ARR}$$

NNTs are easy to interpret but comparisons between NNTs can only be made if the baseline risks are the same. There is no cut-off level for guidance.

NNH is the number needed to harm. This is the number of subjects treated for a length of time for one extra subject to have the adverse event, compared with the control intervention. Smaller NNH values are worse (harm is more frequent).

The NNH:NNT ratio is indicative of the risk/benefit ratio.

Odds ratio

Odds ratio (OR) is an alternative way of comparing how likely events are between two groups.

Odds ratio is the ratio of the odds of having the disorder in the experimental group relative to the odds in favour of having the disorder in the control group.

It is used in cross-sectional studies and case–control studies. In a case–control study, the exposure is often the presence or absence of a risk factor for a disease, and the outcome is the presence or absence of the disease.

$$\text{Odds ratio} = \frac{ad}{bc}$$

- An odds ratio of 1.0 (or unity) reflects exactly the same outcome rates in both groups – that is, **no effect**.
- An odds ratio greater than 1 indicates that the estimated **likelihood** of developing disease is **greater** in the exposed than in the unexposed.
- An odds ratio less than 1 indicates that the estimated **likelihood** of developing the disease is **less** in the exposed than in the unexposed.

Effect size

The effect size is used to compare the results of studies which used different outcome measures. It is calculated for each study by the following equation:

Effect size = (mean in experimental group – mean in control group)/standard deviation of the control group or both groups

It is also known as the 'standardised mean difference'. The larger the value of the effect size, the greater is the impact of the intervention.

Self-assessment exercise 12

1. In a group of 60 patients treated with diclofenac sodium, ten complained of indigestion. What are the risk and odds of developing this side-effect in this group?

2. In a group of 220 patients with heart disease, the risk of death in the first year is 5%. How many patients will die in the first year?

3. In a cohort study, 100 patients were followed up for 20 years. At the start, 56 of the patients had been exposed to asbestos. At the end of the study, of those exposed to asbestos, 20 had lung disease. Of those not exposed, only two had lung disease. Tabulate this information in a contingency table. Calculate the control event rate (CER) and the experimental event rate (EER). Calculate the odds of the outcome in the exposed group and the odds of the outcome in the non-exposed group.

4. A total of 2000 patients with fungal nail infections were randomly allocated to a new topical treatment or placebo (in equal numbers): 66 patients in the placebo group had another infection within 1 month, compared with 21 patients in the treated group. Draw a 2 × 2 table for this information and calculate the following: absolute risk in the treated group (EER), absolute risk in the untreated group (CER), the relative risk (RR), the relative risk reduction (RRR), the absolute risk reduction (ARR) and the number needed to treat (NNT).

5. In a case–control study, 17 patients treated with a new analgesic reported a significant improvement in pain symptoms, whereas four patients did not. In a control group treated with paracetamol, only one of the 20 patients reported a benefit. Calculate the control event rate (CER), the experimental event rate (EER) and the odds ratio (OR).

6. If the relative risk is 1.8 with a 95% confidence interval of 0.7 to 2.1, what does this mean?

COMPARING SAMPLES – THE NULL HYPOTHESIS

Often in research, the results from two or more samples are compared. The researcher is interested in finding out if there are any differences between the groups, as they may highlight an important role for an exposure, investigation or treatment.

To complicate matters, by convention this task is turned on its head, with the researcher assuming that any differences seen are due to chance. The researcher then calculates how likely such differences are indeed due to chance, hoping to show that it is in fact very unlikely.

Step one – the null hypothesis
The **null hypothesis** states that any difference observed in the results of two or more groups is due to chance.

> The null hypothesis is rarely stated in clinical papers and should not be confused with the primary hypothesis. The importance of the null hypothesis lies in the fact that it underpins the statistical tests.

For example, the initial research question may be, 'Does a relationship exist between cannabis smoking and the development of schizophrenia?' The researcher might set up a case–control study to look at past cannabis smoking in a group of schizophrenic patients and matched controls. If there are differences in the exposure to cannabis smoking between the two groups, the researcher dismisses this difference in terms of the null hypothesis, such as 'no relationship exists between cannabis use and schizophrenia.' The researcher then uses statistical tests to calculate the probability that the difference in cannabis smoking prevalence is indeed due to chance and decide whether this probability is large enough to accept, in which case the null hypothesis stands true.

If the results are unlikely to be explained by chance alone, the null hypothesis is rejected and the **alternative hypothesis**, which states that there is a difference not due to chance, is accepted.

Step two – calculating probabilities
Probability is the likelihood of any event occurring as a proportion of the total number of possibilities. The probability of an event varies between 0.0 (never happens) to 1.0 (certain to happen).

Probability in clinical papers is often expressed as the **P value**. P values express the probability of getting the observed results given a true null hypothesis. P values are calculated using statistical methods.

$P < 0.05$ means that the probability of obtaining a given result by chance is less than 1 in 20. By convention, a P value of less than 0.05 is the accepted threshold for **statistical significance** – that is, the null hypothesis can be rejected.

P values greater than 0.05 are non-significant – that is, the null hypothesis is accepted.

This is summarised in **Table 15**. **Table 16** explains the roles of probability in rejecting the null hypothesis in another way. P values may be calculated by several statistical techniques.

$P < 0.05$	$P \geq 0.05$
Less than 1 in 20	Greater than 1 in 20
Results significant	Results non-significant
Null hypothesis is rejected	Null hypothesis is accepted
Evidence of association between variable and outcome	Unproven association between variable and outcome

Table 15 Understanding P values and significance

EVENT	WHAT OTHER PEOPLE SAY	WHAT A RESEARCHER SAYS
Week 1 Dr Cash wins £5 million pounds on the National Lottery	He is as likely as anyone else to win the lottery. His win was due to chance	Null hypothesis: Dr Cash is no more likely to win the lottery than anyone else. The null hypothesis holds true
Week 2 Dr Cash wins the National Lottery again	He is as likely to win as anyone else, even though he won it last week too. He's just incredibly lucky	Null hypothesis: Dr Cash is no more likely to win the lottery than anyone else. The probability of him winning twice in 2 weeks is even more unlikely but it can happen. The null hypothesis holds true
Week 3 Dr Cash wins the National Lottery for the third week in a row	We suspect Dr Cash has not won the lottery three times simply by chance. There is something else going on here to explain these events	The null hypothesis is **rejected** – the association between Dr Cash and the three consecutive lottery wins is not due simply to chance. The probability of this happening is so small that it is not acceptable

Table 16 The role of probability in rejecting the null hypothesis

Step 3 – consider type 1 and type 2 errors

Type 1 errors

The possibility of a type 1 error should be considered with every significant finding.

A type 1 error occurs when the null hypothesis is rejected when it is true. A **false-positive result** has been recorded because a difference is found between groups when no such difference exists. Type 1 errors are usually attributable to bias, confounding or multiple hypotheses testing. The methodology of the study must be scrutinised for these problems.

If a difference is seen between two groups, significance testing must take place to avoid making a type 1 error. P values should be quoted alongside the results. $P = 0.05$ is used as the level of risk we are prepared to take that we will make a type 1 error. The probability of making a type 1 error is equal to P and expressed as α. For example α = 0.05 means that there is only a 5% chance of erroneously rejecting the null hypothesis.

Type 2 errors

The possibility of a type 2 error should be considered with every non-significant finding.

A type 2 error occurs when the null hypothesis is accepted when it is in fact false. The study has returned a **false-negative result** after failing to uncover a difference between the groups that actually exists. This usually happens because the sample size is not large enough and/or the measurement variance is too large.

Type 2 errors can be avoided at the design stage of the study by power calculations that give an indication of how many subjects are required in the trial to minimise the risk of making a type 2 error. The probability of making a type 2 error is represented by β.

Figure 20 and **Table 17** summarise the discussion so far.

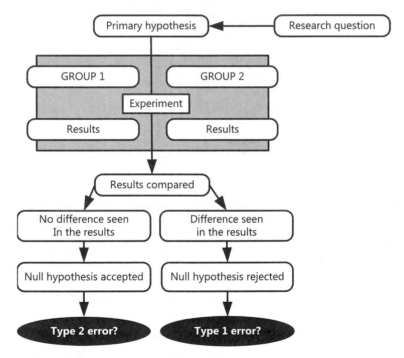

Figure 20 The null hypothesis, P values and type 1 and 2 errors

		NULL HYPOTHESIS	
		True	False
EXPERIMENTAL RESULT	Significant	Type 1 error	Correct
	Not significant	Correct	Type 2 error

Table 17 Summary of type 1 and 2 errors

Sample size and power

The **sample size** for a study is not simply chosen at random. Ideally, a clinical trial should be large enough to detect reliably the smallest possible difference in the outcome measure, with treatment, that is considered clinically worthwhile.

The **power** of a study is its ability to detect a true difference in outcome between the control arm and the intervention arm. This is defined as the probability that a type 2 error will not be made in that study.

Power calculations are made to ensure that the study is large enough to have a high chance of detecting a statistically significant result if one truly did exist. As a general rule, the larger the sample size of a study the more power the study is said to have.

It is not uncommon for studies to be underpowered, failing to detect even large treatment effects because of inadequate sample size. A calculation should be performed at the start of a study to determine the degree of power chosen for that study. For example, a power of 0.8 means there is an 80% probability of finding a significant difference with a given sample size, if a real difference truly did exist, having excluded the role of chance. **A power of 0.8 is generally accepted as being adequate in most research studies.** A study power set at 80% accepts a likelihood of 1 in 5 (ie 20%) of missing such a real difference.

The probability of rejecting the null hypothesis when a true difference exists is represented as $1 - \beta$. Typically, β is arbitrarily set at 0.2. Therefore a study has 80% power (0.8 of a chance) to detect a specified degree of difference at a specified degree of significance.

The key to avoiding type 2 errors is to power the study adequately. In new clinical fields, pilot studies can be carried out to estimate the difference in outcomes between experimental and control groups in order to inform a power calculation. Sometimes studies in progress are double-checked by performing an interim analysis.

A cautious researcher might recruit more subjects than is absolutely required by a power calculation in order to maintain adequate numbers in the trial even if some subjects drop out.

One-tailed versus two-tailed tests

The **alternative hypothesis** is the proposed experimental hypothesis that runs opposite to the null hypothesis. The null hypothesis states that there is no difference between two or more groups. If the null hypothesis is not true, the alternative hypothesis must be true.

Depending on the alternative hypothesis, there may be a choice between one-tailed and two-tailed significance tests.

A **two-tailed test** exists if the alternative hypothesis does not offer a direction for the difference between the groups. One group could do better or worse than the other group.

If the alternative hypothesis does specify a direction, the result is a **one-tailed test**. This may be the case, for example, when comparing a new intervention with a placebo where we would not expect the placebo group to do better. With a one-tailed test, the null hypothesis is modified slightly to state that there is no difference between the groups or the placebo group does better. One-tailed tests are not used often but, when they are, the direction of difference should be specified in advance. The opposite direction is disregarded.

Bonferroni correction

Some research studies include a large number of significance tests. The more tests that are carried out, the more likely it is that a type 1 error will be made. five per cent of significance tests (1 out of 20) are expected to be significant purely due to chance.

The Bonferroni correction safeguards against multiple tests of statistical significance on the same data which might falsely give the appearance of significance. It does this by adjusting the statistical significance level for the number of tests that have been performed on the data. A Bonferroni correction makes it harder to achieve a significant result.

If the Bonferroni correction is excessive, it will increase the risk of making a type 2 error.

Clinical significance

Statistical significance as shown by P values is not the same as **clinical significance**. Statistical significance judges whether treatment effects are explicable as chance findings. Clinical significance assesses whether treatment effects are worthwhile in real life. Small improvements that are statistically significant might not result in any meaningful improvement clinically.

Confidence intervals and significance

A significance result can be deduced from comparing the confidence intervals associated with the summary statistics from two groups. A confidence interval is normally the range of values around a summary statistic in which we are 95% sure the population summary statistic lies.

- When comparing two groups, if the confidence intervals do not overlap this is equivalent to a significant result.

- If the confidence intervals overlap but one summary statistic is not within the confidence interval of the other, the result might be significant.

- If the confidence intervals overlap and the summary statistics are within the confidence interval of the other, the result is not significant.

Self-assessment exercise 13

How would you write the following clinical questions in terms of the null hypothesis?

1. Do patients have problems when they stop paroxetine suddenly?

2. Is atorvastatin more effective than simvastatin at lowering cholesterol levels?

COMPARING SAMPLES – STATISTICAL TESTS

Samples are compared using a variety of statistical tests. Not all statistical tests can be used with all data sets. The determining factors are the number of samples we are comparing, the type of data in the samples and whether the data are **paired** or **unpaired**.

The term 'unpaired' data refers to two groups having different members. Here the selection of the individuals for one group must not be influenced by or related to the selection of the other group. 'Paired' data refers to data from the same individuals at different time points.

Table 18 summarises the statistical tests to use when the types of data collected from the study are the same. As most biological variables are normally distributed, the t-test is one of the most popular statistical tests for comparing two sets of data.

	CATEGORICAL DATA	NON-NORMAL DATA	NORMAL DATA
ONE SAMPLE	Chi-squared test Fischer's exact test (small sample)	Wilcoxon's signed rank test	One-sample t-test
COMPARING TWO GROUPS	Chi-squared test (unpaired) Fisher's exact test (unpaired, small sample) McNemar's test (paired)	Mann–Whitney U test (unpaired) Wilcoxon's matched pairs test (paired)	t-test (paired or unpaired)
COMPARING MORE THAN TWO GROUPS	Chi-squared test (unpaired) McNemar test (paired)	Kruskal–Wallis ANOVA (unpaired) Friedman's test (paired)	ANOVA (paired or unpaired)

Table 18 A summary of statistical tests for comparing samples

Categorical data

Categorical statistical tests involve the use of **contingency tables**, also known as **2 × 2 tables** (Table 19). Remember that disease status positive is always the worst outcome, such as death.

		OUTCOME STATUS		Totals
		positive	negative	
EXPOSURE	positive	a	b	a + b
	negative	c	d	c + d
Totals		a + c	b + d	a + b + c + d

Table 19 The format of a 2 x 2 table

The statistical tests used with categorical data are the chi-squared (χ^2) test (unpaired data) and McNemar's test (paired binary data). For small-sized samples (fewer than five observations in any cell), Fisher's exact test can be used (**Figure 21**).

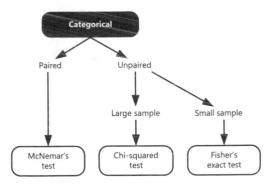

Figure 21 The statistical tests used with categorical data

Degrees of freedom: This is an estimate of the number of independent categories in a particular statistical test or experiment. Dependent categories can be calculated from the independent categories. In the case of a 2 × 2 contingency table, it is the number of ways in which the results in the table can vary, given the column and row totals. A 2 × 2 table has two columns and two rows. If the result in one of the row cells is changed, the result in the other row cell can be calculated. Similarly, if the result in one of the column cells is changed, the result in the other column cell can be calculated. Thus, degrees of freedom is:

(number of rows minus 1) × (number of columns minus 1).

Continuous data

Non-parametric tests, also referred to as 'distribution-free statistics', are used for analysis of non-normally distributed data. The most commonly used tests are, for two independent groups: the Mann–Whitney U test (unpaired groups), Wilcoxon's matched pairs test (for paired data) and, for two or more groups: the Kruskal–Wallis ANOVA (for unpaired data) and Friedman's test (paired data) (**Figure 22**). See **Table 20**.

Non-normally distributed data can either be mathematically transformed into a normal-like distribution by taking powers, reciprocals or logarithms of data values or, alternatively, statistical tests can be used that don't have the assumption of normality.

NON-NORMALLY DISTRIBUTED DATA		
Statistical test	Data	Explanation
Wilcoxon's signed rank test	One sample data	The median of the sample is compared with a hypothetical mean
Mann–Whitney U test	Two unpaired samples	The median of one sample is compared with the median of another sample
Wilcoxon's matched pairs test	Two paired samples	The median of one sample is compared with the median of another sample
Kruskal – Wallis test	Three or more samples of unpaired data	The medians of samples from three or more groups are compared

Table 20 Non-normally distributed data – statistics explained

Parametric tests are used for data that are normally distributed. See **Table 21**.

NORMALLY DISTRIBUTED DATA		
Statistical test	Data	Explanation
One sample t-test	One sample data	The mean of the sample is compared with a hypothetical mean
t-test	Two unpaired samples	The mean of one sample is compared with the mean of another sample
Paired t-test	Two paired samples	The mean of one sample is compared with the mean of another sample
Analysis of variance	Three or more samples of unpaired data	The means of samples from three or more groups are compared

Table 21 Normally distributed data — statistics explained

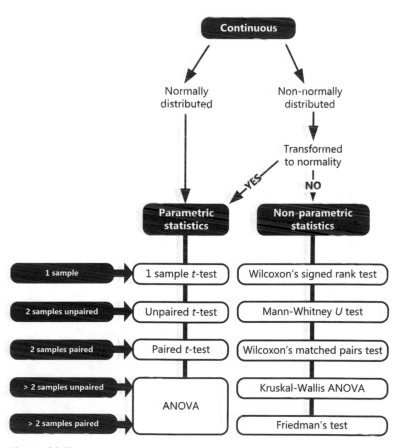

Figure 22 The statistical tests used with continuous data

Advanced statistical analyses

The rest of this chapter tabulates information on advanced statistical analysis. This is provided for reference and not needed in everyday critical appraisal work.

Statistics used for different scales:

	NOMINAL	ORDINAL	INTERVAL	RATIO
Descriptive statistics	Mode	Median	Mean Standard deviation	All
Analytical statistics	Chi-squared test	Percentile	Correlation Regression ANOVA	All

Table 22 Statistics used for different scales

When there is only one outcome variable:

		NUMBER OF MEASUREMENTS PER SUBJECT		
		One	Two	Three or more
OUTCOME VARIABLE	Categorical Binary	Incidence/ prevalence & 95% CI	Kappa McNemar's test	–
	Continuous	Mean, standard deviation & 95% CI Median and IQR One-sample t-test	Intraclass correlation coefficient Mean difference & 95% CI Measurement error Paired t-test	Repeated measures analysis of variance

Table 23

When there is one dependent and one independent variable:

		INDEPENDENT VARIABLE	
		Categorical	Continuous
DEPENDENT VARIABLE (OUTCOME)	Categorical	**Both variables binary:** Chi-squared test Likelihood ratio Logistic regression OR / RR Sensitivity or specificity	**Categorical variable is binary:** Survival analysis
		One or more of the variables has more than two levels: Chi-squared test Kendall's correlation	**Categorical variable is multilevel and ordered:** Spearman's correlation coefficient
	Continuous	**Categorical variable binary:** Independent samples t-test Mean difference & 95% CI	Pearson's correlation Regression
		Categorical variable has three or more categories: ANOVA	

Table 24

Analysis of variance (ANOVA)

This is used to compare the means of three or more groups of continuous or interval scores.

- **A one-way ANOVA** is used when the effect of only one categorical variable (explanatory variable) on a single continuous variable (outcome) is assessed, for example the effect of ethnicity on cholesterol level.

- **A factorial ANOVA / two-way ANOVA** is used when the effects of two or more categorical variables on a single continuous variable are assessed, for example the effect of ethnicity and socioeconomic status on height.

- In **repeated measures ANOVA** the same measure is used on more than one occasion in the same group of patients and it tests the equality of means.

ANOVA also has some multivariate extensions:

- **ANCOVA** (analysis of covariance): This is used when the effects of one or more of the categorical explanatory variables on a single continuous outcome variable are explored after adjusting for one or more continuous variables. These are called covariates. An example is the effects of gender and ethnicity on cholesterol level after adjusting for weight.

- **MANOVA** (multiple analysis of variance): This is used with multiple dependent variables and useful for multiple hypothesis testing.

- **MANCOVA** (multiple analysis of covariance): This is used with multiple dependent and independent variables.

NON-INFERIORITY AND EQUIVALENCE TRIALS

A researcher might pit a new drug against a placebo preparation to illustrate the new drug's efficacy in the management of a condition. However a placebo-controlled trial does not give clinicians the information they want if there is already a treatment available for the condition. In that situation a trial comparing a new drug with the standard drug is more useful.

A researcher can of course set up a trial to assess whether a new drug is better than a standard drug. In such **superiority trials** significance testing is used to determine if there is a difference between the treatments. Superiority studies require large numbers of subjects to ensure adequate power and to minimise type 2 errors because less difference is to be expected when a new treatment is compared with a standard treatment instead of a placebo.

Equivalence

In an **equivalence study** the researcher attempts to show equivalence between drugs. The trial is designed to demonstrate that any difference in outcome between the two drugs lies within a specified range called the equivalence margin or delta. Delta should represent the smallest clinically acceptable difference. Equivalence can be assumed if the confidence interval around the observed difference in effect between the two drugs lies entirely within delta[10].

Non-inferiority

In a **non-inferiority study** the researcher assesses whether a new drug is no worse within a specified margin than the standard drug. If the confidence interval for the difference between the two drugs is not more negative than a prespecified amount, called delta or the non-inferiority margin, then non-inferiority can be assumed[10].

What is the purpose of non-inferiority trials? The answer is that pharmaceutical companies might not need to show that their new drug is better than the standard drug in order to gain market share. For example, if a drug can be shown to be non-inferior and has advantages such as being cheaper or

10   Piaggio G, Elbourne DR, Altman DG, Pocock SJ, Evans SJ. Reporting of noninferiority and equivalence randomized trials: an extension of the CONSORT statement. *JAMA* 2006, 295, 1152–60

causing less adverse effects, the new drug is likely to be prescribed by clinicians. Non-inferiority trials usually require smaller sample sizes and are cheaper and quicker to run than superiority or equivalence trials. Once non-inferiority has been established, further statistical tests can be performed on the data to test for superiority.

Selecting interventions based on class effect

Grouping drugs together depends on the drugs having similar characteristics, which may include chemical structure, pharmacokinetics and pharmacodynamics. A **class effect** exists if the drugs grouped together have similar therapeutic effects and similar adverse effects.

Choosing a drug which belongs to a group and shares a class effect is relatively straightforward because the cheapest option is usually selected.

CORRELATION AND REGRESSION

So far, we have described the data from a single sample, inferred population data from data samples, and compared samples using the null hypothesis. Sometimes it is necessary to establish the nature of the relationship between two or more variables to see if they are associated.

Multivariate statistics enable us to examine the relationships between several variables and make predictions about the data set. There are several methods, depending on the number of variables being examined.

Continuous data can be analysed using correlation and regression techniques.

Correlation

Correlation assesses the **strength** of the relationship between two quantitative variables (**Figure 23**). It examines whether a linear association exists between two variables, X and Y. X is usually the independent variable and Y is usually the dependent variable.

- A **positive correlation** means that Y increases linearly as X increases.
- A **negative correlation** means that Y decreases linearly as X increases.
- **Zero correlation** reflects a complete non-association between the compared variables.

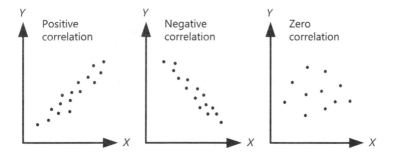

Figure 23 Scatter graphs illustrating three types of correlation

Correlation coefficient

The relationship on a scatter graph can be quantified by the correlation coefficient (r)

- If r is positive, the variables are directly related. As one variable increases, so does the other.

- If r is negative, the variables are inversely related. As one variable increases, the other decreases.

- The value of r varies from -1 to $+1$:

  o if $r = 0$ there is no correlation.

  o the closer r is to 0, the weaker the correlation

  o if $r = -1$ or $r = +1$ there is perfect correlation (all the points fall on a line)

  o the closer r is to -1 or $+1$, the stronger the correlation

  o note that r is not the gradient of the line. The value of r reflects both the direction of any relationship and how tight that relationship is.

Correlation coefficients describe **associations**, ie how two or more variables vary in a related way. Correlation coefficients do not describe causal relationships.

There are different types of correlation coefficients. The correlation coefficient used to describe the relationship between two variables depends on the type of data being compared:

- **Pearson's correlation coefficient, _r_**
  This is a parametric correlation coefficient used to measure the association between continuous variables that are both normally distributed.

  r^2 is the 'coefficient of determination' – an estimate of the percentage variation in one variable that is explained by the other variable.

- **Spearman's rank correlation coefficient, ρ (rho)**
  Used for two ordinal variables or when one variable has a continuous normal distribution and the other is categorical or non-normally distributed.

- **Kendall's correlation coefficient, τ (tau)**
  For correlation between two categorical or non-normally distributed variables.

Regression

Regression determines the nature of the relationship between two or more variables. It involves estimating the best straight line to summarise the association.

The relationship between variables can be represented by the regression line on a scatter graph. The regression line is constructed using a regression equation. The regression equation has predictive value but it does not prove causality.

Simple linear regression

Where there is one independent variable, the equation of the best fit for the regression line is:

$$Y = a + bX$$

Y = value of the outcome variable

a = intercept of the regression line on the y axis

b = regression coefficient (gradient of the regression line), describing the strength of the relationship

X = value of the independent variable

For a given value of X, a corresponding value of Y can be predicted. See **Figure 24**.

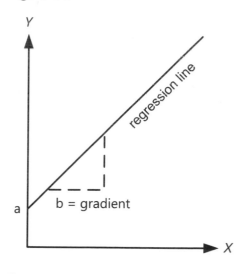

Figure 24 Simple linear regression

Multiple linear regression

A regression model in which the dependent outcome variable is predicted from two or more independent variables is called 'multiple linear regression'. The independent variables can be continuous or categorical.

A measure of association is calculated taking a number of variables into account simultaneously:

$$Y = a + b_1 X_1 + b_2 X_2 + ...$$

$a = Y$ when all the independent variables are zero

b_1, b_2, ... = partial regression coefficients for each independent variable. These are calculated by the **least squares method**. This is usually presented along with a 95% confidence interval and a P value. If $P < 0.05$ or the confidence interval does not contain zero, then the independent variable has a significant influence on the dependent variable

Multiple linear regression is used to assess what effect different variables may have on the study outcome. It is also used to assess the effects of possible confounding factors that may be present in the study.

Logistic regression

This is used where the outcome variable Y is binary in nature and the independents are of any type.

Proportional Cox regression

This is also known as 'proportional hazards regression' and is used to assess survival or an other time-related event.

Factor analysis: This is a statistical approach that can be used to analyse interrelationships among a large number of variables and can be used to explain these variables in terms of their common underlying factors.

Cluster analysis: This is a multivariate analysis technique that tries to organise information about variables so that relatively homogeneous groups, clusters, can be formed.

INTENTION-TO-TREAT ANALYSIS

Scenario 13

Dr Jones returned from his lunch break with renewed vigour. He had just read the conclusion of a trial on the treatment of ear infections in children using a new antibiotic, zapitillin, compared with his usual choice, amoxicillin. In the zapitillin arm, 240 out of 300 children who completed the study improved (80%). In the amoxicillin arm, 300 out of 400 children who completed the study improved (75%). He sent a copy of the paper to his colleague, proposing that zapitillin be first choice in the hospital formulary.

In most studies some of the individuals who are eligible and participate in a trial may not make it to the end of the trial. There are many reasons why such **drop-outs** occur, including early deaths, loss to follow-up (individuals cannot be contacted or have moved out of the study area), voluntary withdrawal from the trial, non-compliance with the trial conditions, and ineligible patients. Some individuals may also not be able to take the treatments offered to them in the trial.

Determining the sample of patients to be analysed is a key step in reporting clinical trials. Ideally, a research paper should account for all its subjects who were eligible and started the trial, explaining the reasons behind some not finishing the trial. In an **intention-to-treat analysis**, all the study participants are included in the analyses as part of the groups to which they were allocated, regardless of whether they completed the study or not. It keeps them in the original groups for the purpose of statistical analysis.

If these patients are not accounted for in the analysis of the results, the results and conclusions might be misleading and important effects of the intervention in terms of, for example, intolerable side-effects, can be lost. Exclusion from the final analysis leads to a bias in interpretation of the results. This is referred to as **attrition bias** (also known as exclusion bias).

Handling missing data

Steps to achieve an intention-to-treat analysis should be considered in both the design and conduct of a trial. Any eligibility errors can be avoided by careful inspection before random allocation. Efforts should be made to ensure minimal drop-outs from treatment and losses to follow-up. In some studies, an active run-in phase is introduced at the start of the study and this can help identify patients who are likely to drop out.

During the trial, continuing clinical support should be available to all participants.

If drop-outs occur in a study, the researcher has to decide how to include these individuals in an intention-to-treat analysis. With luck, some data will have been collected up to the point at which these subjects left the trial. Ideally, data on the primary endpoints are collected after drop out.

- In **last observation carried forward**, the last recorded results of individuals who drop out are carried forward to the end of the trial and incorporated into the final analysis of the results.

- In a **worst-case scenario** analysis, subjects who drop out are treated as non-responders and recorded as having the worst outcome possible. This is the most cautious and pessimistic approach.

- In **imputation**, missing data is substituted to allow the data analysis to proceed. For example, plausible values from similar but complete records might be used to fill in missing values. This is called 'hot-deck imputation'. There are other techniques available. The analysis should take into account the greater degree of uncertainty that is caused by imputation.

- In **sensitivity analysis**, assumptions are made when the missing values are put in. Sensitivity analyses can also be carried out to include different scenarios of assumptions, such as the worst-case and best-case scenarios. Worst-case scenario sensitivity analysis is performed by assigning the worst outcomes to the missing patients in the group who show the best results. These results are then compared with the initial analysis, which excludes the missing data.

- In studies that have many drop-outs, the **drop-out event** itself should be considered as an important endpoint.

It is important to establish whether the reasons drop-outs are no longer taking part are in some way attributable to the intervention. The chance of there being drop-outs should be minimised early on when the study is being planned and during trial monitoring.

Utilisation of 'last observation carried forward' can lead to underestimation or overestimation of treatment effects.

Figure 25 shows the result of treating a depressed patient with an antidepressant. Over the trial, the patient's depressive symptoms improve gradually, such that, at the end of the trial, they were less depressed than at the start.

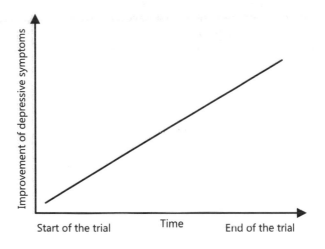

Figure 25 The result of treating a depressed patient with an antidepressant

If a different individual dropped out of the study at an early stage and the last observation was carried forward, the results could underestimate the true effect of the antidepressant, which would have been apparent had the individual completed the trial (**Figure 26**). The risk of making a type 2 error is increased.

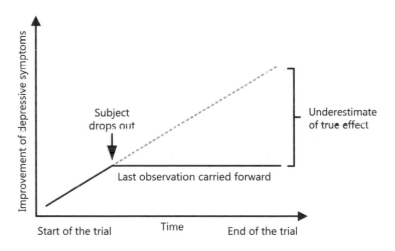

Figure 26 Underestimation of the treatment effect

Overestimation of a treatment effect can occur with last observation carried forward in conditions that normally deteriorate with time.

Figure 27 shows the results of the Mini Mental State Examination (MMSE) score of a dementing individual being treated with an anti-dementia drug. Over the trial, their dementia will progress, but at a slower rate with treatment.

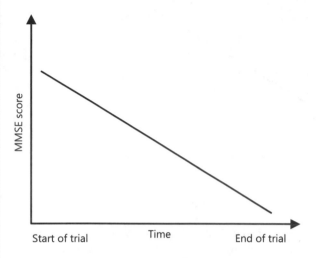

Figure 27 Decline in the Mini-Mental State Examination score

If a different individual drops out of the trial at an early stage, the effects of the anti-dementia drug in delaying the progression of dementia might be over-stated (**Figure 28**). The risk of making a type 1 error is increased.

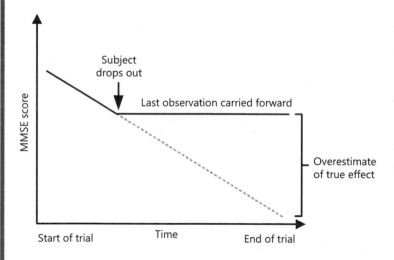

Figure 28 Overestimation of treatment effect

Per-protocol analysis

A per-protocol or on-treatment analysis is an approach used in which data from only those patients who received treatment and complied with the trial protocol are considered in the analysis. The disadvantage of this method is that it can introduce bias related to excluding participants from analysis. A per-protocol analysis tends to enhance any difference between the different groups in a study whereas an intention-to-treat analysis tends to produce more conservative results. Therefore, the intention-to-treat analysis should always be considered as the analysis of choice, and, if necessary, the study could have a secondary analysis using the per-protocol approach.

Scenario 13 revisited

Dr Jones' colleague read the paper too, but came to a different conclusion. He emailed Dr Jones, "I disagree with the conclusions the researchers have drawn. Five hundred patients were enrolled into each arm of the study. I worked out that the results did not take into account the drop-outs in both arms. Intention-to-treat analysis shows that amoxicillin gave better results, with 300 children out of 500 children improving (60%). In contrast, only 240 children improved with zapitillin (48%). I won't be prescribing zapitillin unless the child has an allergy to amoxicillin, but thanks for drawing my attention to the paper."

INTERIM ANALYSIS

Trials may take several months from start to finish. Interim analyses allow researchers to see the results at specific time points before the end of the study. Interim analyses can help to identify flaws in the study design and can help in identifying significant beneficial or harmful effects that might be occurring. This can sometimes result in the study being stopped early for ethical reasons, if it is clear that one group is receiving treatment that is more harmful or less beneficial than another.

There is a potential problem with interim analyses. If multiple analyses are performed, positive findings might arise solely by chance and mislead the researchers into making a type 1 error. Several statistical methods are available to adjust for multiple analyses. Their use should be specified in the trial protocol.

In March 2009 Pfizer stopped a randomised placebo-controlled trial of its drug Sutent (sunitinib) in patients with pancreatic islet cell tumours. The trial began in 2007 and was expected to be completed in 2011. The primary measure of effectiveness was progression-free survival, or time until death or disease progression. An independent data-monitoring committee recommended stopping the trial early after it concluded the drug improved progression-free survival versus placebo. All patients were given the option to continue taking Sutent or be switched from placebo to Sutent.

In April 2009 Pfizer stopped a phase 3 trial comparing its drug Sutent (sunitinib) with Xeloda (capecitabine) in the treatment of advanced breast cancer. The primary endpoint was progression-free survival. An independent monitoring committee found that Sutent was unlikely to prove better as a stand-alone treatment than Xeloda among patients who had not previously benefited from standard treatments.

SYSTEMATIC REVIEWS AND META-ANALYSES

So far, we have been critically appraising individual studies. However, a literature search often reveals many studies with similar aims and hypotheses. Examining one study in isolation may mean that we miss out on findings discovered by other researchers. Ideally, all the studies around one subject area should be collated.

Reviews of articles provide a useful summary of the literature in a particular field. The main flaw with many of these reviews is that they are based on a selection of papers collected in a non-systematic way, so that important research may have been missed.

A **systematic review** attempts to access and review systematically all of the pertinent articles in the field. A systematic review should effectively explain the research question, the search strategy and the designs of the studies that were selected. The results of these studies are then pooled and as a result the evidence drawn from systematic reviews can be very powerful and valuable. The overall conclusions are more accurate and reliable than those of individual studies. Systematic reviews are the gold-standard source of research evidence in the hierarchy of research evidence.

There are four key components to systematic reviews (**Table 25**).

Specifying the research question	Pre-specification of study types Subjects, inclusion, exclusions Intervention/exposure Outcomes Statistical methods
Search strategy	Reproducible Comprehensive Unbiased
Extracting the data	Standardised proforma Study methodology details Assessment of study quality
Interpretation of data	Fixed or random effects models Publication bias for small negative studies Heterogeneity

Table 25 Components of systematic reviews

The QUOROM statement

A conference referred to as the Quality Of Reporting Of Meta-analyses (QUOROM) was held to improve the quality of systematic reviews. This conference resulted in the creation of the QUOROM Statement, which consists of a flow diagram and a checklist of 18 items covering the abstract, introduction, methods and results section of a report of a systematic review of randomised trials[11]. The checklist encourages authors to provide readers with information regarding how the review was set up. The flow diagram provides information about the progress of randomised trials throughout the review process, from the number of potentially relevant trials identified to those retrieved and ultimately included.

Meta-analysis

A meta-analysis is the quantitative assessment of a systematic review. It involves combining the results of independent studies. Meta-analyses are performed when more than one study has estimated the effect of an intervention and when there are no differences in participants, interventions and settings that are likely to affect the outcome significantly. It is also important that the outcome in the different trials has been measured in similar ways. A good meta-analysis is based on a systematic review of studies rather than a non-systematic review which can introduce bias into the analysis.

The results from the studies are combined to produce an overall estimate of effect. As a meta-analysis combines the results of research done on many patients, the analysis has the power to detect small but significant effects. A meta-analysis can provide conclusive evidence for or against an intervention, even when individual studies are inconclusive.

The key steps to remember for a meta-analysis are:

- Synthesis using statistical techniques to combine results of included studies.
- Calculation of a pooled estimate of effect of an intervention, together with its P value and confidence interval.
- Check for variations between the studies (heterogeneity).
- Check for publication bias.
- Review and interpret the findings.

11   Moher D, Cook DJ, Eastwood S, Olkin I, Rennie D, Stroup DF, for the QUOROM Group. Improving the quality of reports of meta-analyses of randomised controlled trials: the QUOROM statement. *Lancet* 1999, 354, 1896–900.

Forest plots

The results of a meta-analysis are presented as a forest plot (or blobbogram) of pooled results. **Figure 29** summarises the components of a forest plot.

The forest plot is a diagram with a list of studies on the vertical axis, often arranged in order of effect or chronological order, and the common outcome measure on the horizontal axis. The outcome measure can be odds or risk ratio, means, event rates, etc. There is a vertical 'line of no effect', which intersects the horizontal axis at the point where there is no difference between the interventions.

The result of each study is shown by a box that represents the point estimate of the outcome measure.

- The area of the box is proportional to the weight each study is given in the meta-analysis. Studies with larger samples sizes and with more precise estimates (ie tighter confidence intervals) are given more weight.

Across each box there is a horizontal line. The width of the horizontal line represents the 95% confidence interval.

- If the horizontal line touches or crosses the line of no effect, either the study outcome is not statistically significant and/or the sample size was too small to allow us to be confident about where the true result lies.

- If the horizontal line does not cross the line of unity, the results are statistically significant.

The overall outcome of the meta-analysis is a diamond shape.

- The centre of the diamond is located at the point estimate of the pooled result.

- The horizontal width of the diamond shape is the 95% confidence interval for the overall result.

- There may be an ascending dotted line from the top point of the diamond.

- In some forest plots the diamond shape is unfilled and the confidence interval is shown as a horizontal line through the diamond. If the confidence interval is narrow, this line might be contained within the diamond.

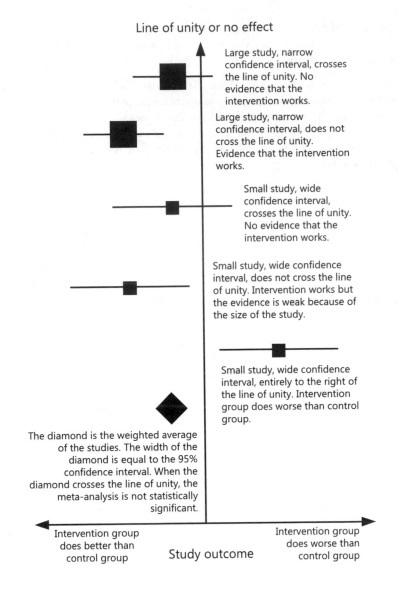

Line of unity or no effect

Large study, narrow confidence interval, crosses the line of unity. No evidence that the intervention works.

Large study, narrow confidence interval, does not cross the line of unity. Evidence that the intervention works.

Small study, wide confidence interval, crosses the line of unity. No evidence that the intervention works.

Small study, wide confidence interval, does not cross the line of unity. Intervention works but the evidence is weak because of the size of the study.

Small study, wide confidence interval, entirely to the right of the line of unity. Intervention group does worse than control group.

The diamond is the weighted average of the studies. The width of the diamond is equal to the 95% confidence interval. When the diamond crosses the line of unity, the meta-analysis is not statistically significant.

Intervention group does better than control group

Intervention group does worse than control group

Study outcome

Figure 29 Understanding a forest plot

Did you know?

The Cochrane Collaboration logo illustrates a forest plot from a systematic review of randomised controlled trials of corticosteroid treatment given to women about to go into premature labour. The forest plot indicates that corticosteroids reduce the risk of babies dying from the complications of immaturity.

HETEROGENEITY AND HOMOGENEITY

Scenario 14

A randomised controlled trial comparing antidepressant treatment against placebo took place in three centres: Manchester, Birmingham and London. The results for Manchester and London were similar. The patients in Birmingham reported remarkably different results, with much bigger improvements in depressive rating scale scores. Before the results of the three centres were combined, a scrutiny of the methodology used in each centre indicated a methodological difference. In Manchester and London, patients were invited to busy outpatient departments to report their progress. In Birmingham, the patients were invited to a hotel suite where they were given tea and cakes while waiting for the researchers. The researchers commented that the difference in results was not due to random chance alone.

Because the aim of the meta-analysis is to summate the results of similar studies, there are tests to ensure that the studies merit combination. Any variation seen to occur between study results can be due to chance or systematic differences or both.

Homogeneity is the term used when studies have similar and consistent results and any observed differences are due to random variation.

When there is more variation than would be expected by chance alone, even after allowing for random variation, this is referred to as **heterogeneity**.

If there is substantial heterogeneity between studies, this can bias the summary effect and the summary statistic is therefore unreliable. By identifying heterogeneity, you can adjust and correct the overall results before producing an overall estimate.

Heterogeneity can occur at different stages. It can occur as differences in the composition of the groups, in the design of the study or in the outcome, eg differences in population characteristics, baseline risks, prescribing effects, clinical settings, methodological differences, outcome measures and, sometimes, unknown differences. It can also occur if the studies are small and the event rate is low so that the results for the groups differ significantly and you cannot rely on the summary estimate.

Clinical heterogeneity occurs when the individuals chosen for two studies differ from one another significantly, making the results of these studies difficult to collate.

Statistical heterogeneity occurs when the results of the different studies differ from one another significantly more than would be expected by chance.

Summary effect size

There are two ways to calculate the effect size to summarise the results for a meta-analysis.

- **Fixed-effects model:** This assumes that there is no heterogeneity between the studies – that is, the trials are all comparable and any differences that may be present are due to the treatments themselves (homogeneity).

- **Random-effects model:** This allows for between-study variations when the pooled overall effect estimate is produced (heterogeneity).

If heterogeneity has been ruled out, a fixed-effects model is used. If heterogeneity does exist, a random-effects model is used. The random-effects model will give wider confidence intervals than fixed-effects models in the presence of significant heterogeneity.

The two types of fixed-effects models for relative risk and odds ratio used to produce a summary statistic are:

- **The Mantel–Haenszel procedure:** The most widely used statistical method for producing the final result of a forest plot. It combines the results of trials, to produce a single-value overall summary of the net effect. The result is given as a chi-squared statistic associated with a P value.

- **The Peto method:** This is for individual and combined odds ratios. This method produces biased results in some circumstances, especially when odds ratios calculated are far from 1.

Methods to test for heterogeneity

- **Forest plot:** This provides visual evidence of heterogeneity if present. Heterogeneity is indicated if the confidence interval of a study does not overlap with any of the confidence intervals of the other studies. If the horizontal lines all overlap to some extent then the trials are homogeneous.

- **Chi-squared statistic:** This tests the null hypothesis that variables estimated from two or more independent samples are the same and that any difference is due to chance alone. Quoted in a meta-analysis, the chi-squared statistic indicates whether there is any variation between the results displayed over and above what would be expected by chance. A low P value (or a large chi-squared statistic relative to its degree of freedom) might provide evidence of heterogeneity. A χ^2 statistic has on average a value equal to its degrees of freedom (ie the number of trials in the meta-analysis minus 1), so a χ^2 statistic of 5 for a set of six trials would provide no evidence of statistical heterogeneity.

- **The Mantel–Haenszel test** can be used to calculate the chi-squared distribution.

- **Z statistic:** If a Z statistic is quoted, this should be associated with a P value or confidence intervals. If $Z > 2.2$, the null hypothesis can be rejected – that is, there is heterogeneity present.

- **Galbraith plot:** A Galbraith plot is useful when the number of studies is small. It is a graph with 1/SE on the x axis and the Z statistic on the y axis. The summary effect line goes through the middle. Heterogeneity is indicated by studies lying a certain number of standard deviations above or below this summary effect line.

Some methods aim to identify homogeneity and as a result can be used to eliminate heterogeneity. For example:

- **L'Abbé plot:** This plots on the x axis the percentage with successful outcome in the control group, and on the y axis the percentage of successful outcome in the experimental group. A diagonal line is drawn between the two axes and above the line represents effective treatment; below the line is ineffective treatment. The more compact the distribution of the points on the graph, the more likely it is that homogeneity is present and the less likely it is that heterogeneity present.

- **Cochran's Q statistic:** Cochran's Q statistic is computed from replicated measurements data with binary responses.

In summary,

If no heterogeneity is found:

- You can perform a meta-analysis and generate a common summary effect measure and

- Decide on what data to combine. Examples of measures that can be combined include:
    - o risk ratio
    - o odds ratio
    - o risk difference

- effect size (z statistic, standardised mean difference)

- *P* values

- correlation coefficient

- sensitivity and specificity of a diagnostic test.

If significant heterogeneity is found:

- You can decide not to combine the data, and

- Find out what factors might explain it, using one of these approaches:

  - graphical methods

  - meta-regression

  - sensitivity analysis

  - subgroup analysis.

Meta-regression analysis

Meta-regression is a method that can be used to try to adjust for heterogeneity in a meta-analysis. It can test to see whether there is evidence of different effects in different subgroups of trials. For example, you can use meta-regression to test whether treatment effects are greater in studies of low quality than in studies of high quality.

Meta-regression analysis aims to relate the size of a treatment effect to factors within a study, rather than just obtaining one summary effect across all the trials. For example, the use of statins to lower cholesterol levels may be investigated by a series of trials. A meta-analysis of these trials may produce a summary-effect size across all the trials. A meta-regression analysis will provide information on the role of statin dosage and its effect on lowering cholesterol levels, helping to explain any heterogeneity of treatment effect between the studies present in the meta-analysis. Meta-regression is most useful when there is high variability in the factor being examined.

Sensitivity analysis

Sensitivity analyses assess how sensitive the results of the analysis are to changes in the way it was done. It allows researchers to see if the results would change significantly if key decisions or underlying assumptions in the set-up and methodology of the trial were changed. If the results are not significantly changed during sensitivity analyses, the researchers can be more confident of the results. If the results do change such that the conclusions drawn will also differ, researchers need to discuss these factors.

PUBLICATION BIAS

Reporting bias is the term applied to a group of related biases that can lead to over-representation of significant or positive studies in systematic reviews. Types of reporting bias include time-lag bias, language bias, citation bias, funding bias, outcome variable selection bias, developed country bias, publication bias and multiple publication bias.

Publication bias

Studies with positive findings are more likely to be submitted and published than studies with negative findings. As a result, smaller studies with negative findings tend to be omitted from meta-analyses, leading to a positive bias in the overall estimate. These positive studies are also more likely to be published in English and more likely to be cited by other authors.

If the results of these small studies differ systematically from those that are included in the systematic review, their exclusion means that the overall results are misleading. The over-representation of positive studies in systematic reviews may mean that the results are biased toward a positive result.

There are several methods available to identify publication bias, including **funnel plots**, the **Galbraith plot** (possible publication bias is indicated by a positive intercept for the regression line, which should pass through the origin), and tests such as **Egger's test** and **Rosenthal's fail-safe N**.

Funnel plots

Funnel plots are scatter plots of treatment effects estimated from individual studies (on the x axis) and some measure of study size on the y axis. The shape of the funnel is dependent on what is plotted on the y axis (**Figure 30**).

The variables on the y axis can include any of the following:

- Standard error
- Precision (1/standard error)
- Sample size
- 1/sample size
- log(sample size)
- log(1/sample size).

The statistical power of a trial is determined by both the sample size and the number of patients that develop the event. This is why the standard error as the measure of study size is a good choice. Also, plotting against precision (1/standard error) emphasises differences between larger studies.

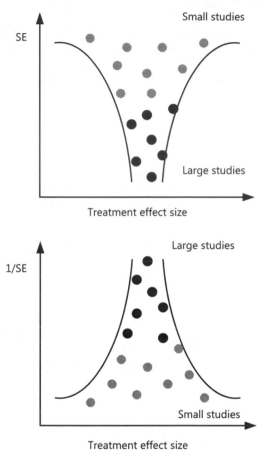

Figure 30 The shape of the funnel plot is dependent on what is plotted on the y axis

Each point on the graph represents one of the studies. Precision in estimating the underlying treatment effect increases as a study's sample size increases. This means that effect estimates from small studies scatter more widely at the open end (widest part) of the funnel. Larger studies have greater precision and provide more similar measures of effect that are nearer to the true effect, and these will lie at the narrow end of the funnel.

Asymmetry of funnel plots

In the absence of bias, the plot therefore resembles a symmetric funnel. If there is publication bias, there will be asymmetry of the open / wide end due to the absence of small negative results (**Figure 31**). Asymmetry can also be due to the tendency for the smaller studies to show larger treatment effects and heterogeneity between trials. The overall estimate of treatment effect from a meta-analysis should be examined closely if there is asymmetry of a funnel plot.

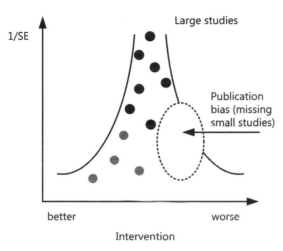

Figure 31 A funnel plot can reveal publication bias

The **'trim and fill'** method can be used with funnel plots to correct for publication bias. First, the number of 'asymmetric' trials on one side of the funnel is estimated. These trials are then removed, or 'trimmed' from the funnel, leaving a symmetric remainder from which the true centre of the funnel is estimated by standard meta-analysis procedures. The trimmed trials are then replaced and their missing counterparts 'filled': these are mirror images of the trimmed trials with the mirror axis placed at the pooled estimate. This then allows an adjusted overall confidence interval to be calculated. Other methods used to detect funnel plot asymmetry include the regression method and the rank correlation approach.

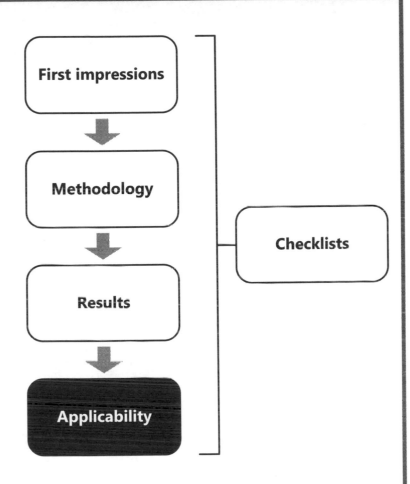

APPLICABILITY

The next stage of critical appraisal is to determine the applicability of the research findings. By this stage you will have decided that the methodology of the study is robust and the results are significant in some way. Some research findings may be of academic interest only whilst others may potentially help your patients. Providing your patients are demographically and clinically similar to the sample population, it may be worth applying the results to your clinical practice, in the expectation that the results on your patients will be similar to the results found in the study population. One could argue that the most useful research is that which can be generalised most easily to a wider population.

Caution needs to be exercised if the results of a study are extrapolated or applied to patients outside the scope of the study. There may not be a linear relationship between variables, which can lead to unexpected benefits and risks to patients who would not have met the inclusion criteria of a study.

The following section on checklists gives further pointers to the applicability of results from different types of studies. The decision to go ahead also depends on your expert knowledge, clinical competency to implement the findings and the availability of resources.

Critical appraisal is but one part of evidence-based medicine. The application and monitoring of any changes to your clinical practice are the final steps in modifying your service to an evidence-based model.

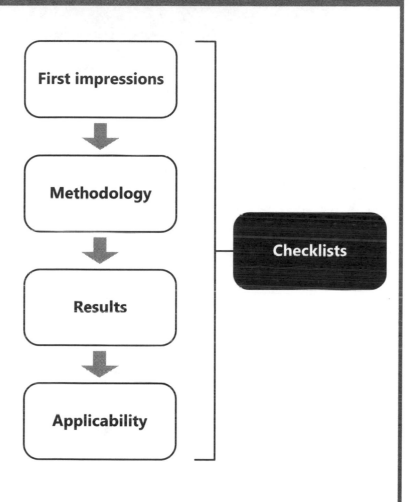

CHECKLISTS

All clinical papers can be understood and critically appraised using the structure that we have described so far. The clinical question and study type are considered before the methodology and results are appraised.

As well as classification of research work by the type of study design used, it can be classified by the subject area of the clinical question. For example, some studies look at aetiological factors; others look at the usefulness of diagnostic tests. Within different clinical areas, there may be specific questions to ask, particularly with regard to the methodology and results. Applicability concerns tend to be the same.

Checklists provide a way to work through the key considerations when critically appraising different study types, by listing the key points in the methodology, reporting of results and applicability. Many institutions have published checklists, but the most highly acclaimed checklists were published in the *Users' guide to the medical literature*, published between 1993 and 2000 in the *Journal of the American Medical Association (JAMA)* by the Evidence-Based Medicine Working Group (see chapter 'Further reading' for references).

The following chapters in this section give a concise overview of the use of checklists that we use in our clinical practice. To avoid duplication, only new terms and concepts are elaborated on.

AETIOLOGICAL STUDIES

Aetiological studies compare the risk of developing an outcome in one or more groups exposed to one or more risk factors (**Figure 32**, **Table 26**). Study types commonly used included case–control and cohort.

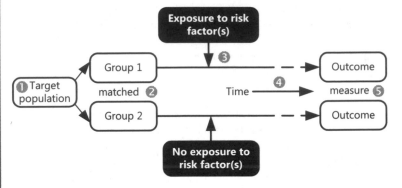

Figure 32 Aetiological studies

METHODOLOGY
Was there a clearly defined group of patients? (1)
Except for the exposure studied, were the groups similar to each other? (2)
Did the exposure precede the onset of the outcome? (3)
Was the follow-up of the subjects complete and of sufficient duration? (4)
Were exposures and clinical outcomes measured in the same way in both groups? (5)

RESULTS
Relative risk in a randomised trial or cohort study
Odds ratio in a case–control study
Precision of the estimate of risk – confidence limits
Is there a dose–response gradient?
Does the association make biological sense?

APPLICABILITY
Are your patients similar to the target population?
Are the risk factor(s) similar to those experienced in your population?
What are your patients' risks of the adverse outcome (number needed to harm)?
Should exposure to the risk factor(s) be stopped or minimised?

Table 26 Aetiological studies checklist

DIAGNOSTIC OR SCREENING STUDIES

A diagnostic study compares a new test for diagnosing a condition with the gold-standard method (**Figure 33, Table 27**).

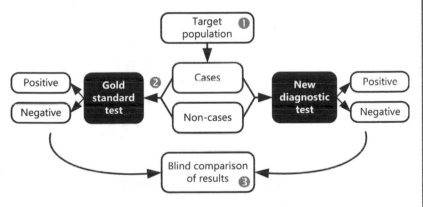

Figure 33 Diagnostic studies

A good test will correctly identify patients with the condition (**true positives**) while minimising the number of patients without the condition who also test positive (**false positives**). Similarly, it will correctly identify patients who do not have the condition (**true negatives**) and minimise the number of patients given negative results when they do have the condition (**false negatives**).

Screening tests look for the early signs of a disease in asymptomatic people so that the disease can be treated before it gets to an advanced stage. The acceptability of false-positive and false-negative results depends in part on the seriousness of the condition and its treatment. A false-positive result causes unnecessary anxiety for the patient and might lead to expensive, unpleasant or dangerous treatments that are not indicated. A false-negative result may lull a patient into a false sense of security and other symptoms and signs of disease may be ignored.

As well as the availability of an accurate diagnostic test, the Wilson and Jungner[12] criteria list other important points to help health organisations decide

12   Wilson J, Jungner G. *Principles and Practice of Screening for Disease.* World Health Organisation. Public Health Papers No. 34, 1968.

whether or not to screen for a disease:

1. The condition sought should be an important health problem.
2. There should be an accepted treatment for patients with recognised disease.
3. Facilities for diagnosis and treatment should be available.
4. There should be a recognisable latent or early symptomatic stage.
5. There should be a suitable test or examination.
6. The test should be acceptable to the population.
7. The natural history of the condition, including development from latent to declared disease, should be adequately understood.
8. There should be an agreed policy on whom to treat as patients.
9. The cost of case-finding should be economically balanced in relation to possible expenditure on medical care as a whole.
10. Case-finding should be a continuing process and not a 'once and for all' project.

Not all diseases are suitable for screening. The UK Screening Portal at http://www.screening.nhs.uk/ lists the current screening programmes in the UK.

METHODOLOGY
Did the patient sample include an appropriate spectrum of patients to whom the test will be applied? (1) Was the gold standard applied regardless of the diagnostic test result? (2) Was there was an independent and blind comparison with a gold standard of diagnosis? (3)
RESULTS
Sensitivity Specificity Positive predictive value Negative predictive value Likelihood ratios Pre-test probability and odds Post-test probability and odds Receiver operating curve
APPLICABILITY
Are your patients similar to the target population? Is it possible to integrate this test into your clinical settings and procedures? Who will carry out the test in your clinical setting and who will interpret the results? Will the results of the test affect your management of the patient? Is the test affordable?

Table 27 Diagnostic or screening studies checklist

Characteristics of the test

The results of the comparison of a diagnostic test with a gold-standard test need to be tabulated in a 2 × 2 table, as shown in Table 28. Note that each subject needs to take **two** diagnostic tests – the gold standard test and the new test. The values of a, b, c and d will either be given or can be deduced from other data given in the results section.

		DISEASE STATUS BY GOLD STANDARD		
		positive	negative	Totals
DISEASE STATUS BY DIAGNOSTIC TEST	positive	a	b	a + b
	negative	c	d	c + d
Totals		a + c	b + d	a + b + c + d

Table 28 2 × 2 tables for the results of diagnostic tests

There are a number of words and phrases used to describe the characteristics of a diagnostic test (**Table 29**). Each of these values should be calculated. A learning aid to help remember the formulae is shown in Figure 34.

TEST CHARACTERISTICS	DESCRIPTION	FORMULA
Sensitivity (true-positive rate)	The proportion of subjects with the disorder (by gold standard) who have a positive result (by new test)	$\dfrac{a}{a + c}$
Specificity (true-negative rate)	The proportion of subjects who do not have the disorder and who have a negative test	$\dfrac{d}{b + d}$
Positive predictive value (PPV)	The proportion of subjects who have a positive test result who do have the disorder	$\dfrac{a}{a + b}$

TEST CHARACTERISTICS	DESCRIPTION	FORMULA
Negative predictive value (NPV)	The proportion of subjects with a negative test result who do not have the illness	$\dfrac{d}{c + d}$
Likelihood ratio for a positive test result (LR+)	How much more likely is a positive test to be found in a person with, as opposed to without, the condition?	$\dfrac{sensitivity}{1 - specificity}$
Likelihood ratio for a negative test result (LR–)	How much more likely is a negative test to be found in a person with, as opposed to without, the condition?	$\dfrac{1 - sensitivity}{specificity}$
Accuracy of a test	The proportion of subjects given the correct result	$(a + d) / (a + b + c + d)$

Table 29 Diagnostic test characteristics

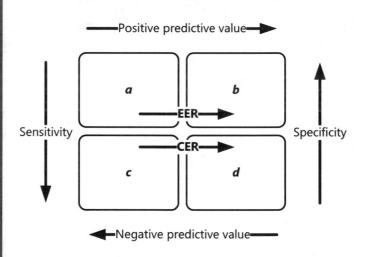

Figure 34 Learning aid for the characteristics of a diagnostic test. For example, the arrow for sensitivity starts at box a and goes over boxes a and c; sensitivity therefore equals a / a + c)

There are also a number of risks and odds that can be calculated for the patient (**Table 30**).

PATIENT RISKS & ODDS	DESCRIPTION	FORMULA
Pre-test probability (equivalent to prevalence)	The probability that a subject will have the disorder before the test result is known	$$\frac{a + c}{a + b + c + d}$$
Pre-test odds	The odds that a subject will have the disorder before the test result is known	$$\frac{\text{pre-test probability}}{1 - \text{pre-test probability}}$$
Post-test odds	The odds that a subject will have the disorder after the test result is known	$\text{pre-test odds} \times R +$
Post-test probability	The probability that the subject will have the disorder after the test result is known	$$\frac{\text{post-test odds}}{\text{post-test odds} + 1}$$

Table 30 Patient risks and odds

Interpreting results

The sensitivity and specificity of a test can be interpreted using the following statements and aides-mémoires:

- **SpPin:** When a highly **sp**ecific test is used a **p**ositive test result tends to rule **in** the disorder.
- **SnNout:** When a highly **sen**sitive test is used, a **n**egative test result tends to rule **out** the disorder.

The sensitivity and specificity describe how abnormality predicts test results. They do not depend on the prevalence of disease.

PPV and NPV give the probability of abnormality for particular test results. However, they depend on the prevalence of the disorder and will change as the disorder becomes rarer in the population:

- PPV will decrease
- NPV will increase
- Post-test probabilities also change.

Likelihood ratios give the probability of abnormality for particular test results and are less likely to change with the prevalence of the disorder. Likelihood ratios are the best indicator of how useful a new diagnostic test is.

The likelihood ratio nomogram (or Fagan's nomogram) enables the post-test probability to be graphically calculated if the pre-test probability and likelihood ratio are known (**Figure 35**). If a line is drawn connecting the pre-test probability of disease and the likelihood ratio, it intersects at the post-test probability of disease when extended to the right.

LR+ > 1   post-test probability > pre-test probability
            Higher LR+ values make it easier to rule in disease

LR+ < 1   post-test probability < pre-test probability
            Lower LR+ values make it easier to rule out disease

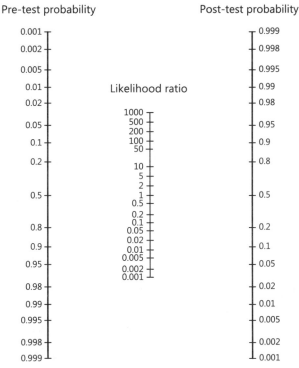

Figure 35 Likelihood ratio nomogram

The performance of a diagnostic test often varies from one clinical location to another and the interpretation of results may also differ. This needs to considered when deciding the applicability of any research findings.

Multiple testing

Serial testing (eg diagnosing HIV – if the first test is positive, another test is done to confirm) increases specificity (true-negative rate).

Parallel testing (eg diagnosing myocardial infarction – history, ECG, enzymes) increases sensitivity (true-positive rate).

Receiver operating characteristic (ROC) curve

There is a threshold with any diagnostic test above which a positive result is returned and below which a negative result is returned. During the development of a diagnostic test, this threshold may be varied to assess the trade-off between sensitivity and specificity.

A good diagnostic test would, ideally, be one that has small false-positive and false-negative rates. A bad diagnostic test is one in which the only cut-offs that make the false-positive rate low have a high false-negative rate and vice versa. To find the optimum cut-off point, a **receiver operating characteristic curve** is used. This is a graphical representation of the relationship between the false-negative and false-positive rates for each cut-off. The plot shows the false-positive rate (1 – specificity) on the x axis and the true-positive rate (sensitivity or 1 – false-negative rate) on the y axis (**Figure 36**).

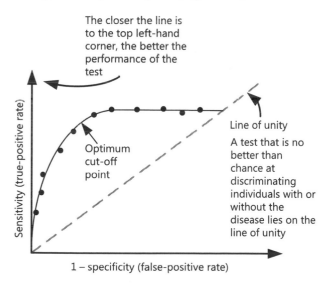

The closer the line is to the top left-hand corner, the better the performance of the test

Optimum cut-off point

Line of unity

A test that is no better than chance at discriminating individuals with or without the disease lies on the line of unity

Sensitivity (true-positive rate)

1 – specificity (false-positive rate)

Figure 36 Receiver operating curve

The **area under the curve** represents the probability that the test will correctly identify true-positive and true-negative results. An area of 1 represents a perfect test, whereas an area of 0.5 represents a worthless test.

The closer the curve follows the left-hand border and then the top border of the receiver operating curve space, the more accurate the test; the true-positive rate is high and the false-positive rate is low. This is the point where the area under the curve is the greatest. The best cut-off point is the point at which the curve is closest to the top left-hand corner.

If two different tests are plotted on the same receiver operating characteristic curve, the test with the curve that lies above the curve of the other test is the best choice.

Self-assessment exercise 14

1. A new test is developed to test for diabetes mellitus. A gold-standard blood test diagnoses 33 people as diabetic out of a study population of 136. The new test diagnoses 34 people as positive, including two people who were not diagnosed by the gold-standard test.
   a. What are the sensitivity, specificity, positive predictive value and negative predictive value for the test?
   b. What are the likelihood ratios for positive and negative test results?
   c. What are the pre-test and post-test probabilities and odds?

TREATMENT STUDIES

Treatment studies compare the effects of a new intervention with those of another intervention (**Figure 37**, **Table 31**). A good intervention will improve the outcome compared with previously available interventions. The improvement may be stated in absolute terms, relative terms or by the number needed to treat (NNT).

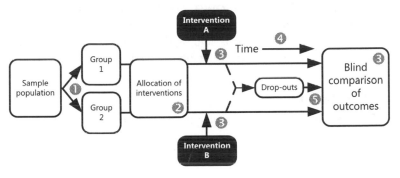

Figure 37 Treatment studies

METHODOLOGY
Was there a clearly focused clinical question and primary hypothesis?
Was the randomisation process clearly explained? (1)
Were the groups similar at the start of the study?
Was concealed allocation used in the allocation of interventions? (2)
Were the groups treated equally apart from the experimental intervention?
Was blinding used effectively? (3)
Was follow-up complete and of sufficient duration? (4)
Was this an intention-to-treat study? (5)

RESULTS
Control event rate
Experimental event rate
Absolute risk reduction / benefit increase
Relative risk reduction / benefit increase
Numbers needed to treat
Precision of the estimate of treatment effect – confidence limits

continued ...

Are your patients similar to the target population?
Were all the relevant outcome factors considered?
Will the intervention help your patients?
Are the benefits of the intervention worth the risks and costs?
Have patients' values and preferences been considered?

Table 31 Treatment studies checklist

Translating NNT to your own patient population

The numbers needed to treat calculated in a study might not directly reflect what will happen in a clinical population, where there are many more factors to consider. There are methods available to estimate the NNT for patients in a clinical setting.

- **Method 1: *F***

  This requires that you estimate your patient's risk compared with the control group from the study. If your patient is twice as susceptible as those in the trial, $F = 2$, etc. The NNT for your patient is simply the trial's reported NNT divided by F, assuming the treatment produces the same relative risk reduction for patients at different levels of risk.

  NNT for your patient = NNT/F

- **Method 2: PEER**

  Alternatively, you could start from an estimate of your patient's risk of an event (patient expected event rate, PEER) without the treatment. This estimate could be based on the study's control group or other prognostic evidence, but you should use your clinical judgement. Multiply PEER by the relative risk reduction or RRR for the study: the result is your patient's ARR, using which NNT for your patient can be calculated:

  $$NNT = 1/(PEER \times RRR)$$

  We assume that the same relative benefit would apply to patients at different levels of risk.

- **Method 3: Bayes' theorem**

  Use a treatment nomogram for Bayes' theorem.

PROGNOSTIC STUDIES

A prognostic study examines the characteristics of the patient (prognostic factors) that could predict any of the possible outcomes and the likelihood that different outcome events will occur (**Figure 38**, **Table 32**). Outcomes can be positive or negative events. The likelihood of different outcomes occurring can be expressed absolutely, relatively or in the form of a survival curve.

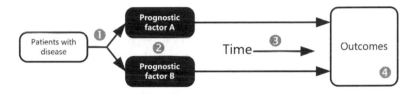

Figure 38 Prognostic studies

Table 32 Prognostic studies checklist

Survival analysis

Survival analysis studies the time between entry into a study and a subsequent occurrence of an event. Originally such analyses were performed to give information on time to death in fatal conditions, but they can be applied to many outcomes as well as mortality.

Survival analysis is usually applied to data from longitudinal cohort studies. There are, however, problems when analysing data relating to the time between one event and another:

- All times to the event occurring will differ, but it is unlikely that these times will be normally distributed.
- Not all subjects may have entered the study at the same time, so there are **unequal observation periods**.
- Some patients may not reach the endpoint by the end of the study. For example, if the event is recovery within 12 months, some patients may not have recovered in the 12-month study period.
- Patients may leave the study early, not experience the event or be lost to follow-up. The data for these individuals are referred to as **censored**.

Both censored observations and unequal observation periods make it difficult to determine the mean survival times, because we do not have all the survival times. As a result, the curve is used to calculate the **median survival time**.

Median survival time

Median survival time is the time from the start of the study that coincides with a 50% probability of survival – that is, the time taken for 50% of the subjects not to have had the event. This value is associated with a P value and 95% confidence intervals.

Kaplan–Meier survival analysis

Kaplan–Meier survival analysis looks at event rates over the study period, rather than just at a specific time point. It is used to determine survival probabilities and proportions of individuals surviving, enabling the estimation of a cumulative survival probability. The data are presented in life tables and survival curves (**Figure 39**).

The data are first ranked in ascending order over time in life tables. The survival curve is plotted by calculating the proportion of patients who remain alive in the study each time an event occurs, taking into account censored observations. The survival curve will not change at the time of censoring, but only when the next event occurs.

Time is plotted on the x axis, and the proportion of people without the outcome (survivors) at each time point on the y axis. A cumulative curve is achieved with steps at each time an event occurs. Small ticks on the curve indicate the times at which patients are censored.

A survival curve can be used to calculate several parameters:

- The **median survival time**, which is the time taken until 50% of the population survive

- The **survival time**, which is the time taken for a certain proportion of the population to survive

- The **survival probability** at a given time point, which is the probability that an individual will not have developed an endpoint event

- It can also be used to compare the difference in the proportions surviving in two groups and their confidence intervals, such as when comparing a control population with an experimental population.

Figure 39 Survival curve

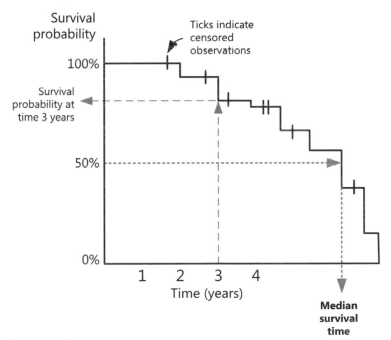

Log rank test
To compare the survival experiences of two or more populations , the proportion of people surviving in each population at any given time point can be

compared. This snapshot does not, however, reflect the total survival experience of the two groups.

The **log rank test** is a better method as it takes the entire follow-up period into account. It is a significance test and helps to decide whether or not to accept the null hypothesis that there is no difference in the probability of survival of the different groups. It does not indicate the size of the difference between the groups, unlike the hazard ratio.

The log rank test is so called because the data are first ranked and then compared with observations and expected outcome rates in each of the groups (similar to a chi-squared test). The log rank test does not take into consideration other variables.

Cox proportional hazards regression

This is the multivariate extension of the log rank test. It is used to assess the impact of treatment on survival or other time-related events and adjusts for the effects of other variables.

Hazard is the instantaneous probability of an endpoint event in a study. It measures the degree of increased and decreased risk of a clinical outcome due to a factor, over a period of time and with various durations of follow up.

Cox proportional hazards regression is used to produce the **hazard ratio**, which is a comparison of the hazard values between two groups. Its interpretation is similar to that of odds ratios and risk ratios. If the hazard ratio is >1, the factor increases the risk of death (or specified outcome). If the hazard ratio is <1, the factor decreases the risk. The hazard ratio is complemented by a *P* value and confidence intervals.

ECONOMIC STUDIES

Resources within the National Health Service are finite. Not every activity can be funded. Economic analyses evaluate choices in resource allocation by comparing the costs and consequences of different actions. They tend to take a wider perspective on healthcare provision than other types of studies, because they do not just focus on whether one intervention is statistically better than another. They aim to discover which interventions can be used to produce the maximum possible benefits.

Economic analyses can be appraised in much the same way as other types of studies (**Table 33**). All direct, indirect and intangible costs and benefits should be included in a good economic analysis. Much of the debate regarding economic analyses tends to focus on the assumptions made in order to calculate monetary values for the use of resources and the consequent benefits. Such assumptions are based on large amounts of information collected from different sources, including demographic data, epidemiological data, socioeconomic data and the economic burden of disease.

METHODOLOGY

Is there a full economic comparison of healthcare strategies?
Does it identify all other costs and effects?
Were the costs and outcomes properly measured and valued?
Were appropriate allowances made for uncertainties in the analysis?
Are the costs and outcomes related to the baseline risk in the treatment population?

RESULTS

Incremental costs and outcomes of each strategy
Cost-minimisation analysis
Cost-effectiveness analysis
Cost–utility analysis
Cost–benefit analysis

APPLICABILITY

Can I use this study in caring for my patients?
Could my patients expect similar outcomes?
Do the costs apply in my own setting?
Are the conclusions unlikely to change with modest changes in costs and outcomes?

Table 33 Economic studies checklist

A sub-discipline of health economics is pharmacoeconomics. This refers to the scientific method that compares the value of one drug with another. A pharmacoeconomic study evaluates the cost (expressed in monetary terms) and effects (expressed in terms of monetary value, efficacy or enhanced quality of life) of a drug.

Examples of input costs
- Direct medical costs – hospitalisations, equipment and facilities, medical and nursing time, drugs and dressings
- Direct non-medical costs – out-of-pocket expenses, time costs, volunteer time
- Indirect costs – productivity changes
- Intangible costs – quality of life, pain and suffering

Examples of output benefits
- Associated economic effects – direct medical savings, direct non-medical savings, indirect savings, intangible savings
- Natural units (health effects) – endpoints, surrogate endpoints, survival
- Utility units (preference-weighted effects) – health status, quality of life

The several types of economic evaluation differ in terms of which consequences they measure.

Cost-of-illness study
This actually is not a true economic evaluation because it does not compare the costs and outcomes of alternative courses of action. It actually measures all the costs that are associated with a particular condition and these can include some of the following:

- Direct costs – where real money is actually changing hands, eg health service use
- Indirect costs – costs that are not directly accountable to a particular function, eg the costs of lost productivity from time off work due to the condition
- Intangible costs – this is the costs associated with the disvalue to a patient of pain and suffering.

Cost consequences study

Outcome of each intervention is measured in different units and as a result you cannot compare the interventions.

Cost minimisation analysis

This analysis is used when interventions are being compared which produce the same beneficial outcome and the benefit is of the same order of magnitude (**Figure 40**).

- Example: The treatment of headache using paracetamol or aspirin.

The analysis simply aims to decide the least costly way of achieving the same outcome.

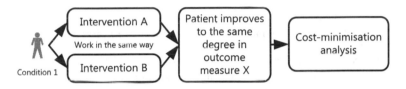

Figure 40 Cost minimisation analysis

Cost-effectiveness analysis (CEA)

This type of analysis is used in situations where the outcome is the same for the alternative interventions but achieved by different mechanisms and to different degrees (**Figure 41**). Therefore the amount of improvement has to be factored in to the economic analysis as well as the cost of the interventions.

- Example: The treatment of back pain using physiotherapy or surgery.

The cost-effectiveness of an intervention is the ratio of the cost of the intervention to the improvement in the outcome measure which is expressed in non-monetary units, such as number of pain-free days. The cost-effectiveness of an intervention is only meaningful when compared with other interventions.

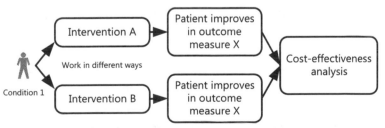

Figure 41 Cost-effectiveness analysis

Cost–utility analysis

A cost–utility analysis is used to make choices between interventions for different conditions in which the units of outcome differ. Cost-utility analysis is better than cost-effectiveness analysis in situations where interventions give outcomes which are not perfect health.

- Example: The treatment of breast cancer using a new drug versus hip replacement surgery.

As the outcomes cannot be directly compared, a common unit, or utility measure, which is indicative of both the quantity and quality of life afterwards is used.

The best known utility measure is the **quality-adjusted life year** or QALY.

QALY = number of extra years of life obtained ×
the value of the quality of life during those extra years

In terms of the quality of life over 1 year, death is equal to 0 QALYs and 1 year of perfect health is 1 QALY. The competing interventions are compared in terms of cost per utility (cost per QALY).

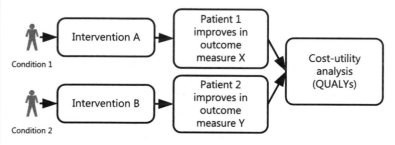

Figure 42 Cost–utility analysis

Example of a cost–utility analysis

A patient needs life-saving treatment.

Intervention A costs £1000 and gives a patient 10 additional years of life with quality of life 0.2. This is equal to 10 × 0.2 = 2 QALYs. The cost of each QALY is £500.

Intervention B costs £2160 and gives a patient 3 additional years of life with quality of life 0.9. This is equal to 3 × 0.9 = 2.7 QALYs. The cost of each QALY is £800.

Over 10 years, intervention B gives 0.7 additional QALYs over intervention A.

There are two ways that this result can influence practice:

1. If the clinician wants to offer the intervention that offers the highest number of QALYs, intervention B is the treatment of choice. The patient may disagree and want to live longer, even if life is harder.

2. If the clinician wants to offer the intervention that offers best value for money for the health service, intervention A is the treatment of choice. The patient may disagree and want a better quality of life, even if life is shorter.

Cost–benefit analysis

This analysis is used to compare the costs and benefits of different treatments for different patient groups by putting a monetary value on the outcome resulting from each alternative intervention. The results for each intervention are expressed as the ratio of economic benefits to costs or as net economic benefit (ie, benefits minus costs). A cost-benefit analysis for a single intervention can be considered on its own so a comparison intervention is not always necessary.

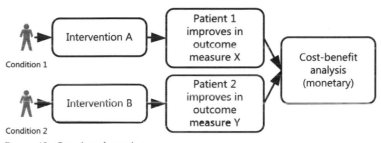

Figure 43: Cost-benefit analysis

Cost-benefit analysis considers the **opportunity cost** of a treatment choice rather than just the direct cost. Using a resource prevents it from being used in some other way. For example, if an intervention is chosen, as well as the direct cost of the intervention itself one has to consider the foregone benefits that may have been gained from choosing an alternative intervention. Only if the costs and benefits associated with the chosen intervention outweigh those of the alternative intervention should the decision to spend go ahead.

Sensitivity analysis

Economic evaluations are models based on assumptions and estimates, and aim to capture and summarise what happens in reality. Sensitivity analysis assists in assessing how robust the conclusions are, considering that there will be a degree of uncertainty about some elements of any economic analysis. It tests the consistency of the results by repeating the comparison between inputs and consequences while varying the assumptions used. The figures are adjusted to account for the full range of possible influences.

A **one-way sensitivity analysis** changes the value of one parameter at a time.

A **multi-way sensitivity analysis** alters two or more parameters simultaneously.

A **probabilistic sensitivity analysis** looks at the effect on the results of an evaluation when the underlying parameters are allowed to vary simultaneously across a range according to predefined distributions. The results it produces are a more realistic estimate of uncertainty. Techniques such as the Monte Carlo simulation have been developed.

QUALITATIVE RESEARCH

In contrast to the objective counting and measuring approach of quantitative research, qualitative research concerns itself with the **subjective** measurement of the processes that underlie behavioural patterns. It can investigate meanings, attitudes, beliefs, preferences and behaviours.

As qualitative research helps doctors to understand people and the social and cultural contexts within which they live, there has been an increasing recognition over recent years of the important role such research can play in the formation and development of medical services. Qualitative methods help to bridge the gap between scientific evidence and clinical practice and help doctors to understand the barriers to using evidence-based medicine, and its limitations in informing decisions about treatment.

A checklist approach can be applied to the evaluation of qualitative research (**Table 34**). As with other types of research, a qualitative study should start with a clearly formulated question that addresses a specific clinical problem and that is amenable to investigation by qualitative methods. Examination of the research question takes place in a natural setting where the patient might normally be.

METHODOLOGY
Did the paper describe an important clinical problem?
Was a qualitative approach appropriate?
How were the participants chosen?
Was the data collection comprehensive and detailed?
Were the data collected in a way that addresses the research issue?
Is there a relationship between researchers and participants that needs consideration?

RESULTS
Was the data analysis sufficiently rigorous?
Were the data analysed appropriately?
Are the results credible and repeatable?
Is there a clear statement of the findings?

APPLICABILITY
Are your patients similar to the patients in this study?
Do the results help you to understand your medical practice and outcomes better?
Does the study help you to understand your relationship with your patients and carers better?

Table 34 Qualitative research checklist

Qualitative data sources include participant observation, focus groups, questionnaires, interviews (structured, semi-structured, in-depth), documents, and the researcher's impressions and reactions. The information collected is about how something is experienced, not measured. The quality and depth of information are important. One strength of qualitative research is that it gets to the heart of the issue and clarifies the fundamental issues.

There are several types of qualitative research methodologies and the **grounded theory** is the most widely used. Unlike quantitative methods, the researcher does not begin with a hypothesis and set out to prove it. Instead, using this approach, a theory is developed to comprehensively explain the findings. The development of the theory begins immediately after the data are collected, rather than being deferred until the end of the study, and continues throughout the entire research process. These data are organised and any trends, associations or causal relationships are examined.

The generalisability of qualitative research is usually limited, and these studies tend to be used for hypothesis generation.

Databases

There are many different databases that cover health and medical subject areas and index research and/or high-quality information resources.

MEDLINE is produced by the National Library of Medicine in the United States (http://www.nlm.nih.gov). It is a major source for biomedical information and includes citations to articles from more than 4000 journals. It contains over 12 million citations dating back to the mid-1960s from international biomedical literature on all aspects of medicine and healthcare. It contains records of journal articles, bibliographic details of systematic reviews, randomised controlled trials and guidelines. There are many organisations that offer access to MEDLINE, with different ways of searching. The key MEDLINE service is offered by the US National Library of Medicine itself, in their PubMed service (www.pubmed.gov).

Current Index to Nursing and Allied Health Literature (CINAHL) is a nursing and allied health database and covers topics such as health education, physiotherapy, occupational therapy, emergency services, and social services in healthcare (http://www.ebscohost.com/cinahl). Coverage is from 1982 to the present, and it is updated bi-monthly.

EMBASE is the European equivalent of MEDLINE, the *Excerpta Medica* database, and is published by Elsevier Science (http://www.embase.com). It focuses mainly on drugs and biomedical literature and also covers health policy, drug and alcohol dependence, psychiatry, forensic science and pollution control. It covers more than 3500 journals from 110 countries and includes data from 1974 onwards. The search engine at www.embase.com includes EMBASE and unique MEDLINE records.

MEDLINE, CINAHL and EMBASE are comprehensive, well-established databases and possess sophisticated search facilities. The size of these databases requires that the searcher first defines the search terms and then refines them to reduce the number of results. Although this can be done by limiting to, for example, publication date, language or review articles only, a more valid way of limiting results is to focus on those articles that are more likely to be of a high quality. This is done by using 'filters'.

NHS Economic Evaluations Database (NHS EED) is a database that focuses on economic evaluations of healthcare interventions. Economic evaluations are appraised for their quality, strengths and weaknesses. NHS EED is available from the website of the Centre for Reviews and Dissemination (http://www.crd.york.ac.uk/crdweb), via the Cochrane Library, via TRIP and via NELH.

The **Turning Research Into Practice (TRIP)** database is a meta-search engine that searches across 61 sites of high-quality information (http://www.tripdatabase.com). Evidence-based publications are searched monthly by experts and indexed fully before being presented in an easy-to-use format with access to full-text articles, medical images and patient leaflets.

Intute, formerly Organising Medical Networked Information (OMNI), is a gateway to hand-selected and evaluated internet resources in health and medicine. It was created by a core team based at the University of Nottingham. Access it at http://www.intute.ac.uk.

APA PsycNET allows users to search **PsycInfo**, an abstract database of psychological literature from the 1800s to the present (http://psycnet.apa.org/). It covers more than 2000 titles, of which 98% are peer-reviewed.

Ovid HealthSTAR contains citations to the published literature on health services, technology, administration and research. It focuses on both the clinical and non-clinical aspects of healthcare delivery.

British Nursing Index (BNI) indexes citations from British and English-language nursing-related journals (www.bni.org.uk).

System for Information on Grey Literature in Europe (SIGLE) is a bibliographic database covering non-conventional literature. This database is no longer being updated.

Google Scholar is a service from the Google search engine (http://scholar.google.com). It provides the ability to search for academic literature located from across the World Wide Web, including peer-reviewed papers, theses, books, abstracts and articles, from academic publishers, professional societies, pre-print repositories, universities and other scholarly organisations. Google has worked with leading publishers to gain access to material that wouldn't ordinarily be accessible to search engines, because it is locked behind subscription barriers. This allows users of Google Scholar to locate material of interest that would not normally be available to them. Google Scholar even attempts to rank results in order of importance.

Evidence-based medicine journals

Several journals, bulletins and newsletters cover evidence-based medicine and clinical effectiveness. Some evidence-based journals, such as the **ACP Journal Club** (www.acpjc.org) published bimonthly by the American College of Physicians and **Evidence-Based Medicine** (http://ebm.bmjjournals.com), scrutinise articles and summarise the studies in structured abstracts, with a commentary added by a clinical expert. These journals cover reviews and choose articles that meet strict selection criteria. **Best Evidence** is a CD-ROM that contains the full text of *ACP Journal Club* and *Evidence-Based Medicine*.

Other examples of newsletters and bulletins include the **Effective Health Care** bulletins (published until 2004, http://www.york.ac.uk/inst/crd/ehcb.htm) and **Bandolier** (http://www.medicine.ox.ac.uk/bandolier/). The latter keeps doctors up to date with literature on the effectiveness of healthcare interventions.

Clinical Evidence (http://www.clinicalevidence.com) is a regularly updated guide to best available evidence for effective healthcare. It is a database of hundreds of clinical questions and answers and is designed to help doctors make evidence-based medicine part of their everyday practice. Topics are selected to cover important clinical conditions seen in primary care or ambulatory settings. There is rigorous peer review of all material by experts, to ensure that the information is of the highest quality. It is updated and expanded every 6 months and is published jointly by *British Medical Journal* journal group and the American College of Physicians.

Evidence-Based Medicine Reviews (EBMR) is an electronic information resource that is available both via Ovid Online (http://www.ovid.com) and on CD-ROM. This database combines three evidence-based medicine sources: the *Cochrane Collaboration's Cochrane Database of Systematic Reviews (CDSR)*, the *Database of Abstracts of Reviews of Effectiveness (DARE)*, ACP Journal Club and the *Cochrane Central Register of Controlled Trials*.

The Cochrane Collaboration

The *Cochrane Library* (http://www.cochrane.org) is an electronic publication designed to supply high-quality evidence to inform people providing and receiving care, and those responsible for research, teaching, funding and administration at all levels. It is a database of the Cochrane Collaboration, an international network of individuals committed to 'preparing, maintaining and promoting the accessibility of systematic reviews of the effects of health care'.

Development and dissemination of guidelines

The **National Library for Health (NLH)** (http://www.library.nhs.uk) provides clinicians with access to the best current know-how and knowledge to support healthcare-related decisions.

The **National Institute for Health and Clinical Excellence (NICE)** was set up as a Special Health Authority for England and Wales on 1 April 1999. It is part of the NHS and it is responsible for providing national guidance on the promotion of good health and the prevention and treatment of ill health (http://www.nice.org.uk).

The **NHS Centre for Reviews and Dissemination (CRD)** is based at the University of York and produces: *Effective Health Care* bulletins (systematic reviews and synthesis of research on clinical and cost-effectiveness); *Effectiveness Matters* bulletins (summaries of systematic reviews); *Systematic Reviews of Research Evidence* (CRD reports).

The **Scottish Intercollegiate Guidelines Network (SIGN)** was formed in 1993 and its objective is to improve the effectiveness and efficiency of clinical care for patients in Scotland by developing, publishing and disseminating guidelines that identify and promote good clinical practice (http://www.sign.ac.uk).

The **National Guideline Clearinghouse (NGC)** is a USA-based public resource for evidence-based clinical practice (http://www.guideline.gov).

Other sources of information

Conference proceedings: Papers given at conferences may give important information on new research either in progress or recently completed. Some trials are only ever reported in conference proceedings. Databases such as the **Conference Papers Index** (http://www.csa.com) hold records and/or abstracts of some proceedings.

Grey literature: This is material that is not published in the standard book or journal formats. It might include reports, booklets, technical reports, circulars and newsletters, and discussion papers.

Citation searching: This involves using reference lists of articles already retrieved or citation indices to trace other useful studies. The **Science Citation Index** (http://scientific.thomson.com/products/sci) allows searching for references using cited authors' surnames.

Hand searching: Journals can be physically examined for their contents. This is time-consuming, but may be viable when the published data from a topic concentrates around a few key journals.

Searching for information

By adopting a sensible search technique, one can dramatically improve the outcome of a search. You can begin by formulating the research question as 'PICO': patient, intervention, comparator and outcome. This will enable you to perform a more structured search for the relevant information and will indicate where the information needs lie. Keywords, similar words or synonyms should then be identified to search terms on the database.

When you start the search, you want to ensure that the search isn't too narrow – that is, that you get as many papers as possible to look at. This is done by **exploding your search**. This means that you can search for a keyword plus all the associated narrower terms simultaneously. As a result, all articles that have been indexed as narrow terms and that are listed below the broader term are included. If too many results are returned, you can refine the search and get more specific results – **focusing your search**. Filters can be used to increase the effectiveness of the search. Subheadings can be used alongside index terms to narrow the search. Indexers can assign up to 20 Medical Subject Headings (MeSH) keywords to an article (see below). These words can also be weighted by labelling them as major headings. These are then used to represent the main concepts of an article. This can help focus the search even more.

Boolean operators are used to combine together keywords in your search strategy.

AND: This is used to link together different subjects. This is used when you are focusing your search and will therefore retrieve fewer references.
For example, 'diabetes' AND 'insulin inhalers' will return items containing both terms.

OR: This is used to broaden your search. You would use OR to combine like subjects or synonyms.
For example, 'diabetes' OR 'hyperglycaemia' will return items containing either term.

NOT: This is used to exclude material from a search.
For example, 'diabetes' NOT 'insipidus' will return items containing the first item and not the second.

Parentheses (nesting) can be used to clarify relationships between search terms.
For example, '(diabetes or hyperglycaemia)' AND 'inhalers' will return items containing either of the first two terms and the third.

A **truncation** symbol at the end of a word returns any possible endings to that word.
For example, 'cardio*' will return 'cardiology', 'cardiovascular', and 'cardiothoracic'. The truncation symbol varies, including a question mark (?), an asterisk (*) and a plus sign (+).

A **wild card** symbol within a word will return the possible characters that can be substituted.

For example, 'wom#n' will return 'woman' and 'women'. Common wild card symbols include the hash (#) and the question mark (?).

Thesaurus: This is used in some databases, such as MEDLINE, to help perform more effective searching. It is a controlled vocabulary and is used to index information from different journals. This is done by grouping related concepts under a single preferred term. As a result, all indexers use the same standard terms to describe a subject area, regardless of the term the author has chosen to use. It contains keywords, definitions of those keywords and cross-references between keywords. In healthcare, the National Library of Medicine use a thesaurus called **Medical Subject Headings (MeSH)**. MeSH contains more than 17 000 terms. Each of these keywords represents a single concept appearing in the medical literature. For most MeSH terms, there will be broader, narrower and related terms to consider for selection. MeSH can also be used by the indexers in putting together entries for Medline databases.

PRESENTING AT A JOURNAL CLUB

Journal clubs are a routine fixture in the academic programmes at teaching hospitals. A successful presentation requires preparation, good presentation skills and clinical relevance for the audience.

Preparation

Different journal clubs take different approaches to the running of the meetings. Some journal clubs are very prescriptive – the clinical paper is already chosen and the doctor has to simply appraise it. Other clubs rely on the doctor to choose a paper of his or her choice. Some clubs ask the doctor to search for and appraise a paper related to a clinical question of interest, such as that which might have been raised by a recent case presentation. However the clinical paper is chosen, preparation has to start well in advance of the presentation.

Ideally, you should distribute the clinical paper to the journal club members at least a week in advance. Most articles are available to download as Adobe Acrobat files from the journal websites; this format maintains their original formatting and provides an excellent original for photocopying. However, be aware of copyright restrictions on distribution. An alternative approach is to publicise the link to the article on the World Wide Web. When you distribute information about your chosen paper, include information on the timing of the journal club and that you will expect everyone to have read the paper before the presentation, which will focus on the critical appraisal of it.

Presentation skills

Nowadays it is not excusable to use anything less than an LCD projector with Microsoft PowerPoint or an equivalent software package for your presentation.

Using PowerPoint

PowerPoint makes it easy to produce great-looking presentations, but unfortunately its flexibility and ease of use also allow doctors to produce presentations that look anything but professional. Use its template features to give your presentation a consistent and professional appearance. Journal clubs are formal affairs, so stick to a dark background colour for your slides, such as blue or black, with lightly coloured text to keep the presentation sober-looking and to aid readability. Avoid patterned backgrounds and fussy templates, which will distract the audience from your presentation. Use a traditional serif typeface, such as Times New Roman, and avoid typefaces that give an informal impression or try to mimic handwriting.

Slide content

Keep each slide brief and to the point. Every slide should have a title and up to five bullet points, which you will expand on during the presentation. Consider using tables or diagrams to summarise information. Avoid abbreviations and acronyms in your presentation, unless your audience is familiar with them. Make sure you double-check your handwriting and grammar. Pay particular attention to the appropriate use of capital letters and punctuation marks. Avoid fancy slide transitions, animations and sound effects.

Delivering the slide show

Dress smartly for your presentation. Leave your mobile phone or pager with a colleague. Arrive early at the journal club, set up your presentation and make sure all the slides appear as designed — don't expect that the technology will always work.

During the presentation, stand to one side of the screen. Talk clearly to the audience, and not too quickly. Make eye contact with different members of the audience for a few seconds at a time. Wireless remote controls, such as the Logitech Cordless Presenter with its built-in timer and laser pointer, enable you to advance through your slides without having to use the keyboard or stand next to the computer. Using such a device can be a liberating experience.

Slides

The organisation of the slides depends on the subject matter. Below is an example of a slide presentation. Resist the temptation to simply read out an abbreviated form of the research paper — your audience has already read it!

SLIDE 1	SLIDE 2
The title of the paper The author(s) of the paper Journal name and date of publication Your name and other details	The clinical question the paper aims to answer The primary hypothesis Comment on the background to this project Comment on originality

SLIDE 3	SLIDE 4
The study design – is it appropriate?	The target population Inclusion and exclusion criteria The sample population The sample size and power calculations

SLIDE 5	SLIDE 6
The randomisation process Concealed allocation	Interventions The blinding process Bias and confounding factors identified

SLIDE 7	SLIDE 8
The outcome measures Validity and reliability of measurements	The null hypothesis Describe the main results

SLIDE 9	SLIDE 10
The statistical methods used Intention-to-treat analysis Completeness of follow-up	Were the aims of the study fulfilled? Are the relevant findings justified? Are the conclusions of the paper justified?

SLIDE 11	SLIDE 12
What is the impact of the paper? Can the results be generalised to your hospital's population?	What do you think of the paper? Summarise the good and bad points What future work can be done? Any questions?

TAKING PART IN AN AUDIT MEETING

The word 'audit' is guaranteed to divide doctors into two camps. On one side are those doctors who leap at the opportunity to improve the services they offer patients. On the other side are those doctors who detest the idea that they should be taken away from clinical work to engage in what they perceive to be a managerial duty. Whatever the attitude towards audit may be, most doctors find themselves doing audit projects because career progression often depends on having evidence of completed audit projects. Importantly, successful audit outcomes depend on a multidisciplinary team approach to ensure practical and timely interventions to improve services. Doctors not engaging in audit do so at their peril and to the detriment of the service as a whole.

Audit meetings usually take place regularly on a monthly basis. To maintain audience interest and continuity, each audit meeting should have on its agenda a mixture of audit presentations, audit protocols for approval and an opportunity for members of the audience to propose audit titles. A rolling agenda should be kept to ensure that teams present their audit projects at the proposal and protocol stages as well as at the end of the first and second cycles of data collection. Only then will audit projects be completed and make a meaningful difference to service provision. Unfortunately it is all too common to see audit projects abandoned after the first data collection due to apathy, doctors moving to different hospitals or a poor understanding of the audit cycle. Each project should have an audit lead who will see the project through to its conclusion.

It is important to distinguish between audits, surveys and research projects. Far too often surveys of service provision are presented as audits where there is no intention of comparing the findings to a gold standard or of repeating the data collection after putting an intervention in place. Other doctors present research projects as a way of sidestepping ethical committees as audit projects do not normally require ethical approval. The chair of the audit meeting needs to keep the meeting focused on audit projects and nothing else.

On the next page is an example of a slide presentation of an audit protocol. Discussions after such presentations tend to focus on the details of the gold standard of service provision to which the local service will be compared. It is imperative that research is done prior to selecting the gold standard to ensure that it is the gold standard! This could mean seeking out national as well as local guidelines on best practice. In the absence of a recognised gold standard, the team may need to make one up or follow the advice of a key opinion leader.

SLIDE 1	SLIDE 2
The title of the audit project The names of the audit lead and participants Date of presentation	A description of the aspect of the service that may need improving

SLIDE 3	SLIDE 4
The gold standard for that part of the service	Details of the first cycle of data collection Who will collect the data and when? What data will be collected?

SLIDE 5	SLIDE 6
The audit tool in more detail	Date of presentation of first data collection and comparison with the gold standard Any questions?

The audit tool is an instrument that facilitates the data collection, which may be done on a retrospective or prospective basis. It is usually a blank form to be filled in with data. The audit tool should be designed to collect only meaningful data and not be over-inclusive. The simpler the audit project, the more likely it is to be completed!

After the first collection of data, the comparison of the local service to the gold standard should be presented at the audit meeting. It is at this point that possible interventions to bring the standard of the local service closer to the gold standard should be discussed with the audience. As far as possible the selected interventions should be pragmatic, likely to succeed and incorporate fail-safe methods.

The completion of the audit cycle requires a final presentation on the second collection of data after the implementation of the agreed interventions. There is, however, no limit to the number of times any aspect of the service can be re-audited.

Done well, audit projects can lead to healthcare environments and procedures that are better suited to the needs of both doctors and patients. It's unlikely that any doctor will complain about that!

WORKING WITH PHARMACEUTICAL REPRESENTATIVES

Doctors differ in their attitudes towards the pharmaceutical industry.

Without a doubt, pharmaceutical companies have revolutionised the practice of medicine. They have invested tremendous amounts in research activity to bring products to the market place that benefit our patients. Without their financial clout, many products would simply never have been in a position to be licensed.

The reputation of some pharmaceutical companies has been tarnished in recent years, however, because of the conflict between their research and marketing departments. The companies exist, after all, to sell products and generate profits. However, as doctors, we should be able to focus our attention on the research work, so that we can decide whether or not our clinical practice can be improved.

The company representative role has evolved over the years in recognition of the changes in the NHS and the acceptance of an evidence-based approach to treatments. In addition to representatives who focus purely on sales, either in primary care or in secondary care, there are those who work on NHS issues with Primary Care Trusts and, in some companies, others that work with outcomes research. Different representatives' objectives will not be the same! An understanding of the roles and responsibilities of pharmaceutical representatives will enable you to maximise the benefits of meeting with them regularly.

The sales representative dissected

Before meeting with you, a pharmaceutical sales representative will know a lot about you. Information about your prescribing habits will have been gleaned from data on dispensed prescriptions. The representative wants to meet you because you are in a position to increase the sales of their company's products. This may be accomplished by more prescriptions, advocating the use of their products to other prescribers, or because you are involved in research that could be favourable to their products.

After the usual greetings and niceties, the focus of the discussion will move to your prescribing habits. The representative wants to gain an insight into how you make decisions about prescribing issues. This involves asking questions about the types of patients you see, the products you prescribe, the reasons for your choice of first-line medications and your experiences of and prejudices against alternative approaches.

The representative will assess your needs in terms of identifying groups of patients in which your outcomes can be improved. They will talk about their company's products and show you evidence of the benefits of prescribing these products for your patients. Sales aids, PowerPoint presentations, promotional literature and clinical papers will magically appear from black briefcases. The effect can be overwhelming, as you are blinded by volumes of impressive data. The representative finishes off the presentation and questioning and asks for some commitment in terms of trying the company's product.

The doctor's viewpoint

Being a passive observer in a meeting with a sales representative is not good use of your time. The representative is usually very knowledgeable about his specialist field and is a potential source of a lot of useful information. You will have your own needs in terms of information you need to be a better doctor, and by identifying these needs to the representative, you can both be in a win–win situation.

There are general questions you can ask to update your knowledge base:

- What is the latest research the company is doing?
- Are there any impending licence changes or new launches?
- Are there any forthcoming NHS initiatives that you should be aware of?
- Which guidelines are in vogue, and who are the key opinion leaders?

If the representative is selling a product to you, you need to focus the discussion on information that will help you to decide whether or not to prescribe the product. Questions you might ask about the data presented can include the following:

- Are these efficacy data or effectiveness data?
- Is the sample population similar to your own?
- What were the inclusion and exclusion criteria?
- What is the comparative treatment? Is it a placebo or is it a head-to-head trial?
- Do the doses used in the study reflect everyday clinical practice?
- What is the absolute risk reduction with the new treatment?
- What is the number needed to treat?
- Are the results statistically significant and clinically significant?
- In which situations should you not prescribe the new treatment?
- Are there any safety data you need to be aware of?

- Why should you not prescribe a competitor product?
- Is this a cost-effective intervention?
- Are there any post-marketing studies in progress?
- Has the drug been through the Drugs and Therapeutics Committee, or has a pharmaceutical advisor been presented with the data?

If you are presented with any graphs, put your analytical skills to the test by looking for marketing tricks in the presentation of data. Examples include the magnification of the y axis to exaggerate differences in comparative results, and the poor labelling of the x axis to hide the short duration of the trial.

Sources of information

Promotional material
The representative can give you approved promotional materials that list product features and benefits. Sales aids help convey important information, such as data on efficacy, safety, tolerability and compliance, comparative data with competitors, health-economic data, the summary of product characteristics and the price.

Clinical papers
Clinical papers provide you with the original data on which promotional material is based. If you prefer to look at the clinical papers, ask the representative to go through the relevant papers or, alternatively, ask for copies to be sent to you. Once you have the paper, you will want to appraise it critically yourself and then arrange to meet with the representative to discuss any issues or questions that you may have. An experienced representative will be able to critique the paper as they use it to sell to you, and point out key details.

Key opinion leaders
You may want to know the opinion of specialists in a field before you prescribe a certain drug. Ask your representative about key opinion leaders and whether they can arrange for you to meet with these people or hear them speak at an appropriate scientific meeting. Alternatively, ask to set up a round-table meeting with you and your colleagues so that you can have an open discussion with the expert about the product and how it would benefit your patients. If you would like to be an advocate for the product, then tell the representative to arrange meetings for you to discuss this with your colleagues.

Data on file

If there is information presented that you are interested in but which has not yet been published, it is usually referenced as 'data on file'. If you would like to see these data, you can request the information and the representative will contact staff in their medical department, who will send this on to you.

Off-licence data

If you have queries that are off-licence, you should let the representative know. They will contact their medical department, and either someone from that department will come and see you or they will send you the requested information. The representative is not allowed to discuss off-licence information.

FURTHER READING

JAMA series

1. Guyatt GH, Sackett DL, Cook DJ, for the Evidence-Based Medicine Working Group. Users' guides to the medical literature. II. How to use an article about therapy or prevention. A. Are the results of the study valid? *Journal of the American Medical Association* 1993, 270, 2598–601.

2. Guyatt GH, Sackett DL, Cook DJ, for the Evidence-Based Medicine Working Group. Users' guides to the medical literature. II. How to use an article about therapy or prevention. B. What were the results and will they help me in caring for my patients? *Journal of the American Medical Association* 1994, 271, 59–63.

3. Jaeschke R, Guyatt G, Sackett DL, for the Evidence-Based Medicine Working Group Users' guides to the medical literature. III. How to use an article about a diagnostic test. A. Are the results of the study valid? *Journal of the American Medical Association* 1994, 271, 389–91.

4. Jaeschke R, Gordon H, Guyatt G, Sackett DL, for the Evidence-Based Medicine Working Group. Users' guides to the medical literature. III. How to use an article about a diagnostic test. B. What are the results and will they help me in caring for my patients? *Journal of the American Medical Association* 1994, 271, 703–7.

5. Levine M, Walter S, Lee H, Haines T, Holbrook A, Moyer V, for the Evidence-Based Medicine Working Group. Users'guides to the medical literature. IV. How to use an article about harm. *Journal of the American Medical Association* 1994, 271, 1615–19.

6. Laupacis A, Wells G, Richardson S, Tugwell P, for the Evidence-Based Medicine Working Group. Users' guides to the medical literature. V. How to use an article about prognosis. *Journal of the American Medical Association* 1994, 272, 234–7.

7. Oxman AD, Cook DJ, Guyatt GH, for the Evidence-Based Medicine Working Group. Users' guides to the medical literature. VI. How to use an overview. *Journal of the American Medical Association* 1994, 272, 1367–71.

8. Drummond MF, Richardson WS, O'Brien BJ, Levine M, Heyland D, for the Evidence-Based Medicine Working Group. Users' guides to the medical literature. XIII. How to use an article on economic

analysis of clinical practice. A. Are the results of the study valid? *Journal of the American Medical Association* 1997, 277, 1552–7.

9. O'Brien BJ, Heyland D, Richardson WS, Levine M, Drummond MF, for the Evidence-Based Medicine Working Group. Users' guides to the medical literature. XIII. How to use an article on economic analysis of clinical practice. B. What are the results and will they help me in caring for my patients? *Journal of the American Medical Association* 1997, 277, 1802–6. Published erratum appears in *JAMA* 1997, 278, 1064.

10. Barratt A, Irwig L, Glasziou P, Cumming RG, Raffle A, Hicks N, for the Evidence-Based Medicine Working Group. Users' guide to medical literature. XVII. How to use guidelines and recommendations about screening. *Journal of the American Medical Association* 1999, 281, 2029–34.

11. Giacomini MK, Cook DJ, for the Evidence-Based Medicine Working Group. Users' guides to the medical literature XXIII. Qualitative research in health care. A. Are the results of the study valid? *Journal of the American Medical Association* 2000, 284, 357–62.

12. Giacomini MK, Cook DJ, for the Evidence-Based Medicine Working Group. Users' guides to the medical literature. XXIII. Qualitative research in health care. B. What are the results and how do they help me care for my patients? *Journal of the American Medical Association* 2000, 284, 478–82.

How to read a paper

A readable and practical series, originally published in the *British Medical Journal*.

1 Greenhalgh T. How to read a paper: the Medline database. *British Medical Journal* 1997, 315, 180–3.

2. Greenhalgh T. How to read a paper: getting your bearings (deciding what the paper is about). *British Medical Journal* 1997, 315, 243–6.

3. Greenhalgh T. How to read a paper: assessing the methodological quality of published papers. *British Medical Journal* 1997, 315, 305–8.

4. Greenhalgh T. How to read a paper: statistics for the non-statistician. I: Different types of data need different statistical tests. *British Medical Journal* 1997, 315, 364–6.

5. Greenhalgh T. How to read a paper: statistics for the non-statistician. II: 'Significant' relations and their pitfalls. *British Medical Journal* 1997, 315, 422–5.

6. Greenhalgh T. How to read a paper: papers that report drug trials. *British Medical Journal* 1997, 315, 480–3.

7. Greenhalgh T. How to read a paper: papers that report diagnostic or screening tests. *British Medical Journal* 1997, 315, 540–3.

8. Greenhalgh T. How to read a paper: papers that tell you what things cost (economic analyses). *British Medical Journal* 1997, 315, 596–9.

9. Greenhalgh T. How to read a paper: papers that summarise other papers (systematic reviews and meta-analyses). *British Medical Journal* 1997, 315, 672–5.

10. Greenhalgh T. How to read a paper: papers that go beyond numbers (qualitative research). *British Medical Journal* 1997, 315, 740–3.

Other useful online resources

The **Critical Appraisal Skills Programme (CASP)** is part of the Public Health Resource Unit based at Oxford (www.phru.nhs.uk/Pages/PHD/CASP. htm). CASP runs training workshops on critical appraisal skills. This site also contains some of their checklists for appraising research.

The **Evidence-Based Medicine Toolkit** is hosted by the University of Alberta (http://www.ebm.med.ualberta.ca). It is an online 'box' of handy tools to help you find, appraise and apply in practice, evidence-based research.

Levels of Evidence and Grades of Recommendation is a ranking system used to rank various study designs in order of evidence-based merit (http://www.cebm.net/levels_of_evidence.asp). Systematic reviews / meta-analyses and well-conducted randomised controlled trials are usually seen as the best form of 'evidence', with research based on the outcome of a case series placed somewhere near the bottom.

The Trent Research and Development Support Unit Research Information Access Gateway (TRIAGE) is a very good list of links to critical appraisal resources compiled by the School of Health and Related Research (ScHARR) at Sheffield (http://www.trentrdsu.org.uk/resources.html). The TRIAGE site provides links to teaching materials, tutorials and articles related to all areas of health research and evidence-based medicine.

ANSWERS TO SELF-ASSESSMENT EXERCISES

Self-assessment exercise 1
Any other significant findings should be regarded as exploratory only, and perhaps give you ideas for further research projects.

Self-assessment exercise 2
1. Case–control study
2. Cohort study
3. Audit
4. Randomised controlled trial
5. Qualitative survey
6. Economic analysis

Self-assessment exercise 3
1. All your patients are given the gold-standard test for meningitis – lumbar puncture. They are also given the blood test that you have developed. The results from the new test are compared with those of the gold-standard test.
2. Your patients will be randomly allocated to one of two groups. One group will receive the new treatment. The other group will receive either a placebo treatment or a pre-existing treatment. After a period of time, the results of the two interventions will be compared.
3. You may choose a case–control study, looking at the risk factors that patients with and without schizophrenia have been exposed to in the past. Alternatively, you may choose a cohort study design, following up people who smoke / don't smoke cannabis to see if they develop schizophrenia.
4. A cohort study of people with and without frozen shoulder are followed up to see if they return to work. Alternatively, one could look at people working and not working and see how many of them have been diagnosed with frozen shoulder.

Self-assessment exercise 4

1. A crossover design requires fewer subjects than a randomised controlled trial because the subjects are their own controls, so they are matched with themselves. However, crossover designs suffer with order effects, historical controls and carry-over effects.

2. Cohort studies observe people who have been exposed to a risk factor to see if they develop an outcome. Case–control studies look at people who already have the outcome and investigate what risk factors they have been exposed to in the past. For investigating rare exposures, cohort studies are better. For investigating rare outcomes, case–control studies are preferred.

3. As a clinician, you should only audit aspects of the service in which you are involved. For example, if you are a doctor in a hospital setting, you should not audit aspects of service provision in a primary care setting. If you did want to audit something that is related to your service but is managed in the primary care setting, it would be acceptable to do a joint project with one of your primary care colleagues.

Self-assessment exercise 5

1. Selection bias: Patients who have suffered cerebrovascular accidents might no longer live at home, or they might be unable to answer the phone.

2. Observation bias: Teenagers may be reluctant to answer questions about drug misuse if questioned by a figure of authority.

3. Selection bias: There will be a concentration of such cases on the ward, resulting in a stronger association than perhaps there is in reality.

4. Observation bias: In the glow of motherhood or after the trauma of childbirth, women may not accurately recall the pain of delivery and the interventions used.

Self-assessment exercise 6

1. Smoking cigarettes

2. Fair skin

3. Smoking

4. Poverty

Self-assessment exercise 7

Inclusion criteria include:

- Adult age group 18–65 years (licence restrictions; criteria for admission to adult wards)
- Diagnosed with schizo-affective disorder
- Hospital inpatient.

Exclusion criteria include:

- Already taking risperidone
- Treatment failure with risperidone in the past ethical consideration
- Comorbid medical and psychiatric conditions
- Coexisting alcohol/drug misuse
- Unable to give informed consent.

Self-assessment exercise 8

1.

    a.   Qualitative, nominal, multicategory

    b.   Qualitative, nominal, binary

    c.   Quantitative, continuous, ratio

    d.   Qualitative, ordinal

    e.   Quantitative, continuous, ratio

    f.   Qualitative, nominal, multicategory

    g.   Quantitative, continuous, ratio

    h.   Qualitative, nominal, multicategory

    i.   Quantitative, continuous, interval

    j.   Qualitative, nominal, multicategory

    k.   Qualitative, ordinal

Self-assessment exercise 9

1.

    a.   mode = 3

    b.   frequencies: value 1 (1), value 2 (2), value 3 (3), value 4 (2), value 5 (1)

    c.   median = 3

    d.   range = 5 − 1 = 4

    e.   mean = $\dfrac{1 + 2 + 2 + 3 + 3 + 3 + 4 + 4 + 5}{9}$ = 3

2.

    a.   median = 15

    b.   range = 100 − 5 = 95

    c.   mean = $\dfrac{10 + 15 + 20 + 100}{5}$ = 30

    d.   The median describes the central tendency of this data set better, because it is less affected by outlying values.

3.

    a.   median = $\dfrac{30 + 35}{2}$ = 32.5

    b.   range = 70 − 5 = 65

    c.   interquartile range:

    i.   split data into quarters: 5, 10, 15 | 20, 25, 30 | 35, 40, 45 | 50, 60, 70

    ii. 1st quartile lies between 15 and 20 = 17.5

    iii. 3rd quartile lies between 45 and 50 = 47.5

    iv.   interquartile range = 47.5 − 17.5 = 30.

4.

    a.   mean = $\dfrac{3 + 13 + 44 + 45 + 51 + 56 + 66 + 75 + 91 + 102}{10}$ = 54.6

    b.   standard deviation = $\sqrt{\dfrac{\sum (x - \bar{x})^2}{n - 1}}$

Calculate $(x - \bar{x})^2$ for all the values	$(3 - 54.6)^2 = 2662.56$
	$(13 - 54.6)^2 = 1730.56$
	$(44 - 54.6)^2 = 112.36$
	$(45 - 54.6)^2 = 92.16$
	$(51 - 54.6)^2 = 12.96$
	$(56 - 54.6)^2 = 1.96$
	$(66 - 54.6)^2 = 129.96$
	$(75 - 54.6)^2 = 416.16$
	$(91 - 54.6)^2 = 1324.96$
	$(102 - 54.6)^2 = 2246.76$

Add all the $(x - \bar{x})^2$ values   8730.4

Divide by n −1 (n = 10) $\dfrac{8730.4}{10 - 1} = 970.04$

Standard deviation is the square $\sqrt{970.04} = 31.15$
root of the result

    c. 95% of observations will lie two standard deviations on either side of the mean.
        mean = 54.6
        standard deviation = 31.15
        2 standard deviations = 31.15 × 2 = 62.3
        range = 54.6 ± 62.3 = −7.7 to 116.9

Self-assessment exercise 10

1.

    a. mean = 16

    b. median = 17

    c. standard deviation = 3.9

    d. standard error = 1.47

2.

    a. mean = 26

    b. median = 17

    c. standard deviation = 28.8

    d. standard error = 10.88

Self-assessment exercise 11

1. Annual incidence rate of lung cancer in the exposed group

    = 4 cases in 100 men in 10 years
    = 0.4 cases in 100 men in 1 year
    = 0.4% annual incidence rate

    Annual incidence rate in unexposed group
    = 1 case in 100 men in 10 years
    = 0.1 case in 100 men in 1 year
    = 0.1% annual incidence rate

    Overall incidence rate
    = 5 cases in 200 men in 10 years
    = 0.5 cases in 200 men in 1 year
    = 0.25 cases in 100 men in 1 year
    = 0.25% annual incidence rate

2. 90 babies delivered every month

    = 1080 babies delivered every year
    1 in 2500 babies affected by cystic fibrosis, ie 0.04%
    0.04% of 1080 = 0.432 babies every year
    = about 4 babies every 10 years

3. 1.3 people in every 100 000 die each year from pancreatitis

    = 780 people in every 60 million die each year from pancreatitis
    = 15 people in every 60 million die each week from pancreatitis

4. 85 000 people with multiple sclerosis in a population of 60 million
    = 141 people with multiple sclerosis in a population of 100 000
    prevalence rate = 141 per 100 000

5. Effects on prevalence
    a. increased
    b. decreased
    c. decreased
    d. decreased

Self-assessment exercise 12

1. risk $= \dfrac{10}{60} = 0.166 = 16.6\%$

    odds $= \dfrac{10}{50} = 0.2$

2. 5% of 220 = 11

3.

		LUNG DISEASE		
		positive	negative	Totals
EXPOSURE TO ASBESTOS	positive	20	36	56
	negative	2	42	44
Totals		22	78	100

$$CER = \frac{2}{44} = 4.5\%$$

$$EER = \frac{20}{56} = 35.7\%$$

Odds in exposed group $= \frac{20}{36} = 0.56$

Odds in non-exposed group $= \frac{2}{42} = 0.05$

4.

		FUNGAL NAIL INFECTION		
		positive	negative	Totals
GIVEN NEW TREATMENT	positive	21	979	1000
	negative	66	934	1000
Totals		87	1913	2000

Absolute risk in the treated group (EER) $= \frac{21}{1000} = 0.021 = 2.1\%$

Absolute risk in the untreated group (CER) $= \frac{66}{1000} = 0.066 = 6.6\%$

Relative risk $= \frac{0.021}{0.066} = 0.32 = 32\%$ (an improvement)

$$\text{Relative risk reduction} = \frac{0.066 - 0.021}{0.066} = 0.68$$

$$\text{Absolute risk reduction} = 0.066 - 0.021 = 0.045$$

$$\text{The number needed to treat} = \frac{1}{0.045} = 22$$

5.

		PAIN SYMPTOMS IMPROVED		
		positive	negative	Totals
GIVEN NEW ANALGESIC	positive	17	4	21
	negative	1	19	20
Totals		17	24	41

$$CER = \frac{1}{20} = 0.05$$

$$EER = \frac{12}{21} = 0.81$$

$$\text{Odds ratio} = \frac{17 \times 19}{4 \times 1} = 80.75$$

6. You can be 95% sure that the true relative risk lies between the values 0.7 and 2.1. Alternatively, you can be 5% sure that the true relative risk is less than 0.7 or greater than 2.1. Note that the range of the relative risk contains the null hypothesis value of 1, so the relative risk result is not statistically significant.

Self-assessment exercise 13

1. Paroxetine is not associated with discontinuation symptoms.

2. Atorvastatin is as effective at lowering cholesterol levels as simvastatin
   or
   Atorvastatin is no more effective than simvastatin at lowering cholesterol levels.

Self-assessment exercise 14

1. First draw a 2 × 2 table

		DISEASE STATUS BY GOLD STANDARD		
		positive	negative	Totals
DISEASE STATUS BY NEW TEST	positive	32	2	34
	negative	1	101	102
Totals		33	103	136

$$\text{Sensitivity} = \frac{32}{33} = 0.97$$

a. $$\text{Specificity} = \frac{101}{103} = 0.98$$

$$\text{Positive predictive value} = \frac{32}{32 + 2} = 0.94$$

$$\text{Negative predictive value} = \frac{101}{1 + 101} = 0.99$$

b. $$\text{Likelihood ratio for a positive test result} = \frac{0.97}{1 - 0.98} = 48.5$$

$$\text{Likelihood ratio for a negative test result} = \frac{1 - 0.97}{0.98} = 0.03$$

c. $$\text{Pre-test probability} = \frac{32 + 1}{32 + 2 + 1 + 101} = 0.24$$

$$\text{Pre-test odds} = \frac{0.24}{1 - 0.24} = 0.31$$

$$\text{Post-test odds} = 0.31 \times 48.5 = 15.03$$

$$\text{Post-test probability} = \frac{15.03}{15.03 + 1} = 0.94$$

A FINAL THOUGHT

It is never an easy task to initiate, plan and complete a research project. It requires dedication, hard work and a willingness to work long hours, which are often unpaid and unrecognised. Few researchers aim deliberately to publish poor-quality research. More often than not, limitations in trial design and conduct are due to a lack of resources, ethical considerations or simply that pragmatic solutions have to be found to enable the research project to take place.

The attainment of critical appraisal skills allows doctors to evaluate the quality of research papers. Such skills should be used, not only to find flaws in clinical papers, but also to comment positively on the good points. Taking a balanced approach will ensure that all research, good and bad, generates ideas for future projects. It is this endless cycle of thinking, questioning and doing that has brought us so far. The journey is far from complete.

In 1676, Isaac Newton wrote to a fellow scientist, acknowledging the work of others in his own research:

> If I have seen further, it is by standing on the shoulders of giants.

INDEX

2 x 2 tables (contingency tables) 82–3, 86, 95, 135

absolute risk (AR) 84
absolute risk reduction (ARR) 84
abstracts 5
accuracy (validity) 57, 58–9, 136
adaptive randomisation 50
adverse drug reactions 15
aetiological studies (causation) 8, 19, 132
allocation (randomisation methods) 48–52
allocation of resources see economic analysis
alternative hypothesis 87, 92
see also null hypothesis
alternative-form reliability 61
analysis of variance (ANOVA) 97, 99–100
applicability of results 32, 127
AR (absolute risk) 84
ARR (absolute risk reduction) 84
article structure 5–6, 22–3
attrition bias 37, 107
audit 24, 166–7, 176
average (mean) 71

Bayes' theorem 142
Berkson (admission) bias 36
bias in study design/execution 34–8, 107, 176
prevention of 46–55
bias in study publication 121–3
blinding 52, 53–4
block randomisation 49
BNI (British Nursing Index) database 158

Bonferroni correction 92

case–control studies 17–18, 47
case reports 15
case series 15–16
CASP (Critical Appraisal Skills Programme) 174
categorical (qualitative) data 65, 66, 67
comparative statistics 94, 95, 98, 99
descriptive statistics 69
causation studies (aetiology) 8, 19, 132
CER (control event rate) 84
chi-squared (χ^2) test 95, 118–19
CI (confidence interval) 76, 93, 115
CINAHL (Current Index to Nursing and Allied Health Literature) 157
citations 3–4, 160
class effects 102
Clinical Evidence (BMJ/ACP) 159
clinical question, assessment of 7–9
clinical significance 93
clinical trials
regulatory phases 30–1
see also study design
cluster analysis 106
cluster randomisation 50
cluster sampling 33
Cochrane Collaboration xiii, 116, 159
Cochran's Q statistic 119
cohort studies 18–19, 47
composite endpoints 56
concealed allocation 51–2
concurrent validity 58
conference proceedings 160

confidence interval (CI) 76, 93, 115
conflicts of interest 5–6
confounding factors 39–43, 47, 49, 176
consent 49
CONSORT statement 22–3
construct validity 59
content validity 59
contingency tables 82–3, 86, 95, 135
continuous data 65–6, 67
    comparative statistics 94, 96–7, 98, 99–100, 103–6
    descriptive statistics 69–77, 178–9
control event rate (CER) 84
control matching 47
controlled trials 20, 22–3
convenience sampling 33
convergent validity 58
correlation 103–4
cost–benefit analysis 151
cost consequences studies 149
cost-effectiveness analysis 8, 25, 149
cost minimisation analysis 149
cost-of-illness studies 148
cost–utility analysis 150–1
covariance 42, 100
Cox proportional hazards regression 106, 146
CRD see NHS Centre for Reviews and Dissemination
Critical Appraisal Skills Programme (CASP) 174
Cronbach's α statistic 61
cross-sectional studies 14, 25
crossover trials 20–1

databases 157–8
degrees of freedom 95
diagnostic purity bias 36, 46
diagnostic studies 8, 133–40, 183
discriminant validity 58
distribution 69–73, 178–9

double-dummy technique 54
drop-outs (missing data) 107–11

ecological studies 14
economic analysis 25, 147–52, 158
EER (experimental event rate) 84
effect size 86, 115, 118–20
effectiveness xv–xvi, 14, 31
efficacy xv–xvi, 20
EMBASE database 157
endpoints 56–62
epidemiological studies 78–81, 180
equivalence studies 101
ethics 45, 112
evidence-based medicine xiii–xvi, 159
Evidence-Based Medicine Toolkit 174
exclusion (attrition) bias 37, 107
experimental event rate (EER) 84
experimental studies 20–3, 30–1, 141–2
experts 5, 170

F value (NNT analysis) 142
face validity 59
factor analysis 106
false-negative results (type 2 errors) 90–2, 109, 133, 139
false-positive results (type 1 errors) 10, 89–90, 92, 109–10, 133, 139
financial (economic) analysis 25, 147–52, 158
Fisher's exact test 95
fixed-effects model 118
forest plots 115–16, 118
frequency 69
funnel plots 121–3

Galbraith plots 119
Google Scholar 158
grey literature 158, 160
grounded theory 154

guidelines 160

Hawthorne effect 37
hazard/hazard ratio 106, 146
heterogeneity of study results 117–20
hierarchy of evidence 28–9, 174
historical control bias 36
homogeneity of study results 117–20
hospital standardised mortality ratio 79
'how to read a paper' 173–4
hypotheses
    null/alternative 87–93, 182
    primary/secondary 10

immediacy index 4
impact factors in journal evaluation 3–4
imputation 108
inception cohorts 33
incidence 78–9, 81, 180
incremental validity 59
information sources 131, 157–62, 170–4
intention-to-treat analysis 107–11
interim analysis 112
internet-based resources 157–60, 174
    search strategies 161–2
interquartile range 70–1
inter-rater reliability 60–1
interval scales 67, 98
interviewer (ascertainment) bias 36
intra-class correlation coefficient 61
intra-rater reliability 61
Intute 158

Journal of the American Medical
    Association (JAMA) 172–3
journal clubs 163–5
journals
    article structure 5–6, 22–3
    evaluation of quality of 3–4
    of evidence-based medicine

159, 172–3
    on-line resources 157–9

Kaplan–Meier survival analysis 144–5
kappa statistic (κ) 60–1
Kendall's correlation coefficient (τ) 104
Kruskal–Wallis test 96
kurtosis 73

L'Abbé plots 119
'last observation carried forward'
    method 108–10
likelihood ratio 136, 138, 183
linear regression 105–6
log rank tests 145–6
logistic regression 106
longitudinal studies 143–6

Mann–Whitney U test 96
Mantel–Haenszel procedure 42, 118, 119
masking (blinding) 52, 53–4
matching of subjects 47
McNemar's test 95
mean 71
measurement of data
    scales 67–8, 177
    types of data 65–6
median 70
median survival time 144, 145
Medical Subject Headings (MeSH) 162
MEDLINE database 157
membership bias 36
meta-analysis 25, 114–16
    heterogeneity of data 117–20
    publication bias 121–3
meta-regression 120
minimisation (adaptive
    randomisation) 50
missing data 107–11
mode 69

morbidity rates/ratios 79
mortality rates/ratios 78–9, 81, 180
multiple linear regression 106
multivariate analysis 42, 100,
    103–6, 146

n-of-1 trials 21
National Guideline Clearinghouse
    (NGC) (USA) 160
National Institute for Health and
    Clinical Excellence (NICE) 160
    guidelines on hierarchy of
    evidence 29
National Library for Health (NLH)
    160
negative predictive value (NPV) 136,
    137–8, 183
Neyman (incidence/prevalence) bias
    36
NHS Centre for Reviews and
    Dissemination (CRD) 160
    guidelines on hierarchy of
    evidence 28–9
NHS Economic Evaluations Database
    (NHS EED) 158
NICE see National Institute for Health
    and Clinical Excellence
NNH (number needed to harm) 85
NNT (number needed to treat) 85,
    142
nominal scales 67, 98
non-inferiority studies 101–2
non-normal distribution 69–71, 94,
    96, 104
non-parametric tests 96, 104
normal distribution 71–2, 94, 96–7,
    104
NPV (negative predictive value) 136,
    137–8, 183
null hypothesis 87–93, 182
number needed to harm (NNH) 85
number needed to treat (NNT) 85,
    142

observation bias 36–7, 38, 53–4,
    176
observational analytical studies
    17–19, 47, 85
observational descriptive studies
    15–16
odds 82, 86, 137, 180, 181
odds ratio (OR) 85, 118
off-license data 171
one-tailed tests 92
online resources 157–60, 174
    search strategies 161–2
open trials 20
opinion leaders 5, 170
OR (odds ratio) 85, 118
ordinal scales 67, 98
outcomes (endpoints) 56–62
outliers 70
Ovid HealthSTAR database 158

P values 87–93
paired/unpaired data 94, 97
parametric tests 96–7, 104
Pearson's correlation coefficient (r)
    104
peer review 3
PEER value 142
per-protocol analysis 111
performance bias 35, 36
periodicals see journals
Peto method 118
pharmaceutical company
    representatives 168–71
pharmacoeconomics 148
PICO (analysis of clinical questions)
    8–9
placebos 44–5, 54
populations in a study see sample
    population
positive predictive value (PPV) 135,
    137–8, 183
post-marketing surveillance studies
    31
power of a study 91–2, 122

PowerPoint presentations 163–5
PPV (positive predictive value) 135, 137–8, 183
pragmatic trials 14
precision (reliability) 57, 60–2, 122
predictive validity 58
presentation skills 163–5
prevalence 80, 81, 180
primary hypothesis 10
probability (risk) 82–6, 180–2
    in diagnostic tests 137, 138, 183
    significance testing 87–93
prognostic studies 8, 143–6
proportional hazards regression 106, 146
prospective studies 18 19, 47
PsycInfo database 158
publication bias 35, 121–3

qualitative (categorical) data 65, 66, 67
    comparative statistics 94, 95, 98, 99
    descriptive statistics 69, 178–9
qualitative research 24–5, 153–4
quality-adjusted life year (QALY) 150
quantitative data 65–6, 67
    comparative statistics 94, 96–7, 98, 99–100, 103–6
    descriptive statistics 69–77, 178–9
quasi-random allocation 49–50
QUOROM statement 114

r (correlation coefficient) 104
random sampling 33
random-effects model 118
randomisation methods 48–52
randomised controlled trials (RCTs) 20, 22–3
ratio scales 67, 98
recall bias 37
receiver operating characteristic

(ROC) curves 139–40
regression 105–6
relative risk (RR) 84
relative risk reduction (RRR) 84
reliability (precision) 57, 60–2, 122
reporting bias 35, 121–3
research pathway for drug development 30–1
resource allocation see economic analysis
response bias (observational) 37
response bias (sampling) 36
retrospective (case–control) studies 17–18, 47
retrospective cohort studies 19
risk (probability) 82–6, 180–2
    in diagnostic tests 137, 138, 183
    significance testing 87–93
ROC (receiver operating characteristic) curves 139–40
RR (relative risk) 84
RRR (relative risk reduction) 84

sales representatives, dealing with 168–71
sample population
    allocation of 48–52
    selection of 32–3, 35–6, 41, 46–7, 177
    size of 91–2
sampling bias 36
sampling error 74–6, 122
scale types 67–8, 98, 177
screening (diagnostic) studies 8, 133–40, 183
SD (standard deviation) 71–2
SE (standard error) 74–5, 122
selection bias 35–6, 38, 46, 51–2, 176
sensitivity analysis 108, 120, 151–2
sensitivity in diagnostic tests 135, 137, 139, 183

service provision, assessment of 24–5, 166–7, 178
SIGLE (System for Information on Grey Literature in Europe) database 158
SIGN (Scottish Intercollegiate Guidelines Network) 160
significance testing 87–93
skewed data 69–71, 73
Spearman's rank correlation coefficient (ρ) 104
specificity in diagnostic tests 135, 137, 139, 183
split-half reliability 61
standard deviation (SD) 71–2
standard error (SE) 74–5, 122
standardisation 42
statistical significance 88, 93
stratification 33, 42
stratified randomisation 49
study design 55
    bias and 34–8, 46–55, 176
    clinical trial phases 30–1
    confounders 40–3
    hierarchy of evidence 28–9
    placebos 44–5, 54
    subjects see sample population
    types of 13–27, 175–6
subgroup analysis 10
subjects see sample population
superiority trials 101
surrogate endpoints 56
surveys 24–5, 153–4
survival analysis 106, 144–6
systematic reviews 25, 113–14

meta-analysis 114–23
systematic sampling 33

t-tests 97
target population 32
test–retest reliability 60
thesauri 162
treatment studies 8, 20–3, 30–1, 141–2
TRIAGE website 174
trim and fill method 123
TRIP (Turning Research Into Practice) database 158
two-tailed tests 92
type 1 errors (false positives) 10, 89–90, 92, 109–10, 133, 139
type 2 errors (false negatives) 90–2, 109, 133, 139

unpaired/paired data 94, 97
unpublished data 121, 160, 171

validity (accuracy) 57, 58–9, 136

websites 157–60, 174
    search strategies 161–2
Wilcoxon's matched pairs test 96
Wilcoxon's signed rank test 96
worst-case scenario analysis 108

Yellow Card scheme 15

z score/Z statistic 72, 119